Endocrine Disorders During Pregnancy

Endocrine Disorders During Pregnancy

Editors

Sarita Bajaj MD DM
Past President, Endocrine Society of India
Consultant Endocrinologist
Director-Professor and Head of Medicine
Moti Lal Nehru Medical College
Allahabad, UP, India

Rajesh Rajput MD DM (Endocrinology) FICP FIACM FIMSA
Senior Professor and Head
Department of Medicine VI and Endocrinology
Pt BD Sharma Post Graduate Institute of Medical Sciences
Rohtak, Haryana, India

Jubbin J Jacob MD DNB
Associate Professor and Head
Endocrine and Diabetes Unit, Department of Medicine
Christian Medical College
Ludhiana, Punjab, India

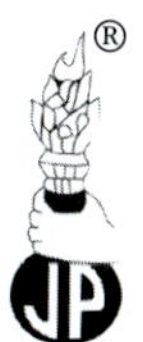

JAYPEE BROTHERS MEDICAL PUBLISHERS (P) LTD.

New Delhi • London • Philadelphia • Panama

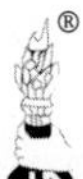

Jaypee Brothers Medical Publishers (P) Ltd.

Headquarters
Jaypee Brothers Medical Publishers (P) Ltd
4838/24, Ansari Road, Daryaganj
New Delhi 110 002, India
Phone: +91-11-43574357
Fax: +91-11-43574314
Email: jaypee@jaypeebrothers.com

Overseas Offices
J.P. Medical Ltd
83 Victoria Street, London
SW1H 0HW (UK)
Phone: +44-2031708910
Fax: +02-03-0086180
Email: info@jpmedpub.com

Jaypee-Highlights Medical Publishers Inc.
City of Knowledge, Bld. 237, Clayton
Panama City, Panama
Phone: + 507-301-0496
Fax: + 507-301-0499
Email: cservice@jphmedical.com

Jaypee Brothers Medical Publishers, Ltd
The Bourse
111 South Independence Mall East
Suite 835, Philadelphia, PA 19106, USA
Phone: + 267-519-9789
Email: joe.rusko@jaypeebrothers.com

Jaypee Brothers Medical Publishers (P) Ltd
17/1-B Babar Road, Block-B, Shaymali
Mohammadpur, Dhaka-1207
Bangladesh
Mobile: +08801912003485
Email: jaypeedhaka@gmail.com

Jaypee Brothers Medical Publishers (P) Ltd
Shorakhute, Kathmandu
Nepal
Phone: +00977-9841528578
Email: jaypee.nepal@gmail.com

Website: www.jaypeebrothers.com
Website: www.jaypeedigital.com

Inquiries for bulk sales may be solicited at: jaypee@jaypeebrothers.com

Endocrine Disorders During Pregnancy / Eds. Sarita Bajaj, Rajesh Rajput, Jubbin J Jacob
First Edition: **2013**

ISBN 978-93-5025-573-5

Printed at: Sanat Printers, Kundli

Contents

Contributors *vii*
Preface *ix*
Acknowledgments *xi, xiii*

1. **Endocrine Physiology in Pregnancy** **1**
Sarita Bajaj

2. **Pregnancy and Diabetes Mellitus** **12**
Rajesh Rajput

3. **Iodine Metabolism in Pregnancy** **24**
Maria Thomas, Jubbin J Jacob

4. **Hypothyroidism and Pregnancy** **36**
Rajesh Rajput

5. **Thyrotoxicosis in Pregnancy** **46**
Sudeep K, Jubbin J Jacob

6. **Parathyroid Disorders During Pregnancy** **58**
Rajesh Rajput

7. **Endocrinology of Hyperemesis Gravidarum** **66**
Roopa Verghese, Jewel Jacob, Jubbin J Jacob

8. **Hypertension and Pregnancy** **79**
Rajesh Rajput

9. **Vitamin D and Pregnancy** **88**
Sarita Bajaj

10. **Bone Disorders and Pregnancy** **96**
Sarita Bajaj, Afreen Khan

11. **Pituitary Disorders in Pregnancy** **105**
Simon Rajaratnam, Geeta Chacko

12. **Adrenal Disorders in Pregnancy** **118**
Sarita Bajaj

13. **PCOS and Pregnancy** **131**
Sarita Bajaj

14. **Obesity and Pregnancy** **139**
Sarita Bajaj, Afreen Khan

15. **Fetal Origins of Endocrine Disease** **151**
Senthil Vasan K, Veena Nair, Nihal Thomas

Index *163*

Contributors

EDITORS

Sarita Bajaj MD DM
Past President, Endocrine Society of India
Consultant Endocrinologist
Director-Professor and Head of Medicine
Moti Lal Nehru Medical College
Allahabad 211 001, UP, India

Rajesh Rajput MD DM (Endocrinology) FICP FIACM FIMSA
Senior Professor and Head
Department of Medicine VI and Endocrinology
Pt BD Sharma Post Graduate Institute of Medical Sciences
Rohtak 124 001, Haryana, India

Jubbin J Jacob MD DNB
Associate Professor and Head
Endocrine and Diabetes Unit, Department of Medicine
Christian Medical College
Ludhiana 141 008, Punjab, India

CONTRIBUTING AUTHORS

Geeta Chacko MBBS MD
Professor-Neuropathology
Department of Neurological Sciences
and Pathology
Christian Medical College
Ida Scudder Road, Vellore 632 004
Tamil Nadu, India

Jewel Jacob MD
Department of Critical Care
The Duncan Hospital
East Champaran District
Raxaul 845 303
Bihar, India

Sudeep K MD DNB
Assistant Professor
Endocrinology Unit
Department of Medicine
Father Muller Medical College and Hospital, Kankanady
Mangalore 575 002
Karnataka, India

Afreen Khan MD
Senior Resident
Department of Medicine
Moti Lal Nehru Medical College
Allahabad 211 001
UP, India

Veena Nair MBBS MD Dch PDCC
Senior Research Associate
Department of Endocrinology
Diabetes and Metabolism
Christian Medical College
Ida Scudder Road, Vellore 632 004
Tamil Nadu, India

Simon Rajaratnam MD DNB MNAMS FRACP PhD
Professor and Head
Endocrinology Unit-2
Christian Medical College
Ida Scudder Road
Vellore 632 004
Tamil Nadu, India

Maria Thomas MD
Associate Professor
Department of Biochemistry
Christian Medical College
Ludhiana 141 008, Punjab, India

Nihal Thomas MBBS MD MNAMS DNB FRACP FRCP
Professor and Head
Department of Endocrinology
Diabetes and Metabolism
Vice-Principal (Research)
Christian Medical College
Ida Scudder Road, Vellore 632 004
Tamil Nadu, India

Senthil Vasan K MBBS (PhD)
Department of Molecular Medicine and Surgery, Karolinska Institutet
Stockholm, S17176, Sweden
Department of Endocrinology
Diabetes and Metabolism
Christian Medical College and Hospital
Ida Scudder Road, Vellore 632 004
Tamil Nadu, India

Roopa Verghese MD
Department of Obstetrics and Gynecology
The Duncan Hospital
East Champaran District
Raxaul 845 303
Bihar, India

Preface

The burden of endocrine disorders during pregnancy is enormous whether one considers the magnitude of the population afflicted, the impact on the lives of affected women, the rendered morbidity, or the economic toll taken by it. Our healthcare system fails to adequately meet the needs of patients with chronic diseases, in general and endocrine diseases, in particular. Referrals of patients to endocrinologists are infrequent, and there are not sufficient number of these specialists. Additionally, there is under-representation of the subject in medical schools' curricula when compared to the burden of these diseases. This is particularly the case when it is appreciated that virtually, all medical specialities are impacted.

Healthcare professionals must not only diagnose and treat problems in the most appropriate and efficient way but also educate the general public at large to prevent these disorders. Education is achieved by assimilating information from many sources. This book has tried to cover a broad base of scientific knowledge and clinical expertise in an integrated way that aims to be accessible to the non-specialist. This edition has a total of 15 chapters, including endocrine physiology and iodine nutrition in normal pregnancy. All endocrine glands-related disorders in relation to pregnancy are covered. Polycystic ovarian syndrome (PCOS) and pregnancy, obesity and pregnancy, and endocrinology of hyperemesis gravidarum have been discussed in detail. Long-term outcomes of pregnancy on the fetus and fetal programming is appropriate for concluding the title. Every chapter has been written to ensure that it reflects the cutting edge of medical knowledge and practice, pitched at a level of detail to meet the needs of practising physicians.

We hope that the information gathered in this text will help both caregivers and patients. So, if this book facilitates reading, proves useful in everyday work, allows you to browse with ease, read with pleasure, and learn without pain, our goal will be achieved.

Sarita Bajaj

Rajesh Rajput

Jubbin J Jacob

Acknowledgments

I wish to acknowledge and thank the following for their help in the writing of *Endocrine Disorders During Pregnancy*.

First I wish to thank my colleagues Dr Rajesh Rajput and Dr Jubbin J Jacob for assisting the progress of the book throughout its many stages of development. The valuable inputs of Dr Maria Thomas, Dr Sudeep K, Dr Roopa Verghese, Dr Jewel Jacob, Dr Simon Rajaratnam, Dr Geeta Chacko, Dr Senthil Vasan K, Dr Veena Nair, Dr Nihal Thomas are much appreciated. I am indeed indebted to all the contributors whose expertise knowledge and scholarship leap from every page.

Next in line are the team members of M/s Jaypee Brothers Medical Publishers (P) Ltd., New Delhi, India for providing support and encouragement in making this book possible. I am particularly indebted to Dr Madhu Choudhary for her sound advice. Dr Mrinalini Bakshi, Mr DC Gupta, and Mr Manoj Kumar deserve to be lauded for their valuable inputs.

My sincere thanks to Dr Afreen Khan who has been instrumental in the shaping of this book.

I am indebted to the contributors whose expertise knowledge and scholarship leap from every page.

Words are insufficient to express my gratitude to my husband, Dr AK Bajaj, who fuelled my ability, remained my guiding force, and allowed me to concentrate on writing.

We all take immense pride in our efforts to produce this diligently crafted book.

Sarita Bajaj

Acknowledgments

When it comes to acknowledgement or gratitude, one is filled up with such revered feelings that suddenly words start to lose their meaning, sentences become feeble to bear the burden, and dictionary flounders to express the gratitude for those helping hands, who brought the present work on horizon.

I wish to acknowledge the help and support of Dr Sarita Bajaj, Dr Jubbin J Jacob, and all the contributing authors in the writing of *Endocrine Disorders During Pregnancy.*

I owe special thanks to the entire team of M/s Jaypee Brothers Medical Publishers (P) Ltd., New Delhi, India and especially, to Dr Madhu Choudhary, for providing timely help and support in the shaping of this book.

Last, but not the least, with deepest sense of love and gratitude, I am thankful to my wife Dr Meena and my children, Siddhant and Vasundhara, who helped me out in most difficult times by their constant encouragement, advice, love, and care, which added to the stores of my energy to complete this work in time.

Lastly, I take immense pleasure in introducing this book to all those, who are involved in care of pregnant women suffering from one or the other endocrine problems.

Rajesh Rajput

1

Endocrine Physiology in Pregnancy

Sarita Bajaj

INTRODUCTION

Pregnancy is a dynamic and an anabolic state. The endocrinological processes of gestation comprise various endocrine and metabolic changes as a consequence of physiological modifications at the fetoplacental boundary between the mother and the fetus. The neuroendocrine events and their timing in the placental, fetal, and maternal compartments are critical for initiation and maintenance of pregnancy, for growth and development of fetus, as well as for parturition.[1,2] Within several weeks of conception, a new endocrine organ, the placenta, is formed that secretes hormones which affect the metabolism of all nutrients.[1]

The endocrine system is amongst the earliest system that develops in the fetus, and remains functional from early intrauterine existence to the prime of life. The fetal endocrine system, to some extent, relies on the precursors secreted by either placenta or in the mother's body for its regulation. As the fetus develops, its own endocrine system matures and eventually becomes more independent to prepare it to cope with extrauterine life.[2]

THE PLACENTA AND ITS HORMONAL ROLE

The development of human placenta is as uniquely intriguing as the embryology of the fetus. The fetus, during its brief intrauterine existence, depends on placenta for pulmonary, hepatic, and renal functions. The placenta, through its unique anatomical association with the mother, accomplishes these functions.[3]

The corpus luteum and placenta secrete hormones, which maintain pregnancy and influence metabolism.[1] The placenta functions partly as a hypothalamic-pituitary-end organ-like entity with stimulatory and inhibitory feedback mechanisms to regulate dynamic factors affecting fetal growth and development under a variety of conditions.[2]

The production of steroid and protein hormones by human trophoblasts is greater in amount and diversity than that of any single endocrine tissue in the whole mammalian physiology.[3] Placental steroidogenesis takes place in the syncytiotrophoblast, and synthesis and secretion of estrogen and progesterone increase throughout pregnancy in concert with an increase in the trophoblast mass.[4]

The human placenta also synthesizes an enormous amount of protein and peptide hormones as much as 1 g of human placental lactogen (HPL) every 24 hours, massive quantities of human chorionic gonadotropin (hCG), adrenocorticotropic hormone (ACTH), growth hormone variant (GH-V), parathyroid hormone-related protein (PTH-rP), calcitonin, relaxin, inhibins, activins and atrial natriuretic peptide, as well as a variety of hypothalamic-like releasing and inhibiting hormones, such as thyrotropin releasing hormone (TRH), gonadotropin releasing hormone (GnRH), corticotropin releasing hormone (CRH), somatostatin, and growth hormone-releasing hormone (GHRH) (Table 1-1).[3]

Progesterone

After 6–7 weeks of gestation, small amounts of progesterone are produced in the ovary.[5] After about 8 weeks, the placenta replaces the ovary as the source of progesterone and continues its production in such a way that there is a gradual increase in the levels throughout the remaining pregnancy. By the end of pregnancy, maternal levels of progesterone are 10–5,000 times than those in nonpregnant women, depending on the stage of the ovarian cycle. The daily production rate of progesterone in late, normal, singleton pregnancy is about 250 mg.[3] The trophoblast preferentially use maternal low-density lipoprotein (LDL) cholesterol for progesterone biosynthesis. Progesterone appears to have multiple functions during pregnancy, the most important being preparation of the uterus for implantation and maintenance of the pregnancy.

TABLE 1-1

Steroid Production Rates in Nonpregnant and Near-term Pregnant Women

Steroid	*Production rates (mg/24 hours)*	
	Nonpregnant	*Pregnant*
17-Estradiol	0.1–0.6	15–20
Estriol	0.02–0.1	50–150
Progesterone	0.1–40	250–600
Aldosterone	0.05–0.1	0.250–0.600
Deoxycorticosterone	0.05–0.5	1–12
Cortisol	10–30	10–20

Adapted from Maternal Physiology. In: Cunningham FG, Leveno KJ, Bloom SL, Hauth JC, Gilstrap LC III, Wenstrom KD, Editors. Williams Obstetrics, 22nd edition, McGraw-Hill Publications; 2007.

Progesterone also serves as an important substrate for fetal adrenal glucocorticoid and mineralocorticoid synthesis and maintenance of myometrial quiescence, possibly through inhibition of prostaglandin formation. A possible role for the high concentrations of progesterone present at the trophoblast-decidua junction is suppression of cell-mediated rejection of the fetus, which expresses paternal antigens, by maternal T lymphocytes.[6]

Estrogen

The placenta produces huge amount of estrogen using blood-borne steroidal precursors from the maternal and fetal adrenal glands. Near term, normal human pregnancy is a hyperestrogenic state of major proportions. The amount of estrogen produced each day by syncytiotrophoblast during the last few weeks of pregnancy is equivalent to that produced in 1 day by the ovaries of not less than 1,000 ovulatory women. The estrogen levels continually increase as pregnancy progresses and terminate abruptly after parturition.[3] By the seventh week, more than 50% of estrogen entering the maternal circulation is produced by the placenta. During pregnancy, estrogen has several actions as stated below:[4]

- Enhances receptor-mediated uptake of LDL cholesterol, which is important for normal placental steroid production
- Increases uteroplacental blood flow
- Increases endometrial prostaglandin synthesis
- Prepares the breasts for lactation.

Human Chorionic Gonadotropin

hCG, the so-called pregnancy hormone, is a glycoprotein with biological activity very similar to luteinizing hormone (LH), both of which act via the plasma membrane LH–hCG receptor. hCG is produced almost exclusively in the placenta but is also synthesized in fetal kidney, and a number of fetal tissues may produce the β-subunit or intact hCG molecule.[7] The intact hCG molecule is detectable in the plasma of pregnant women about 7–9 days after the midcycle surge of LH that precedes ovulation. Thus, it is likely that hCG enters maternal blood at the time of blastocyst implantation. Blood levels increase rapidly, doubling every 2 days, with maximal levels being attained at about 8–10 weeks of gestation. The best-known biological function of hCG is the so-called *rescue and maintenance of function of the corpus luteum*, i.e., continued progesterone production.[3]

Human Placental Lactogen

HPL is synthesized and secreted by the syncytiotrophoblast and is detected in the maternal serum between 20 and 40 days of gestation.[8] Maternal plasma concentration rises steadily until about 34–36 weeks, and this rise is linked mainly to the placental mass. The serum concentration reaches higher levels in late pregnancy (5–15 g/mL) than that of any other known protein hormone. HPL has putative actions in a number of important metabolic processes. These include:[9]

- Maternal lipolysis and an increase in the levels of circulating free fatty acids, thereby, providing a source of energy for maternal metabolism and fetal nutrition
- An anti-insulin or "diabetogenic" action leading to an increase in maternal levels of insulin, which favors protein synthesis and provides a readily available source of amino acids for transport to the fetus
- A potent angiogenic hormone, it also may play an important role in the formation of fetal vasculature.

PITUITARY GLAND

The maternal anterior pituitary gland enlarges by an average of 36% during pregnancy primarily because of a tenfold increase in lactotroph size and number. This enlargement results in an increase in height and convexity of the pituitary on magnetic resonance imaging (MRI). There are reduced number of somatotrophs and gonadotrophs and no changes in corticotrophs or thyrotrophs.[10] The posterior pituitary gland diminishes in size during pregnancy.[11] The maternal pituitary gland is not essential for maintenance of pregnancy.[3]

The marked increase in estrogen levels during pregnancy enhances prolactin synthesis and secretion, and maternal prolactin serum levels increase in parallel with the enlargement of the lactotrophs (Figure 1-1). At term, the mean serum prolactin concentration is 207 ng/mL (range 35–600 ng/mL), in contrast to a mean of 10 ng/mL in nonpregnant premenopausal women.[12] The principal function of maternal serum prolactin is to ensure lactation.[13] Prolactin levels return to the baseline level of nonpregnancy approximately 7 days after delivery in the absence of breastfeeding. With breastfeeding, the basal prolactin levels remain elevated for several months but gradually decrease; however, with suckling, there is a brisk rise in prolactin levels within 30 minutes.[10]

Growth hormone (GH) levels in maternal serum remain unchanged throughout pregnancy, although the source of immunoreactive GH during gestation does change. Relaxin, secreted by the corpus luteum of pregnancy and estrogen stimulate GH secretion during early pregnancy.[14] During the first trimester, GH is secreted predominantly from the maternal pituitary gland and concentrations in serum and amniotic fluid are within nonpregnant values of 0.5–7.5 ng/mL.[15] As early as 8 weeks, GH-V secreted from the placenta becomes detectable.[16] By about 17 weeks, placenta is the principal source of GH-V secretion.[17]

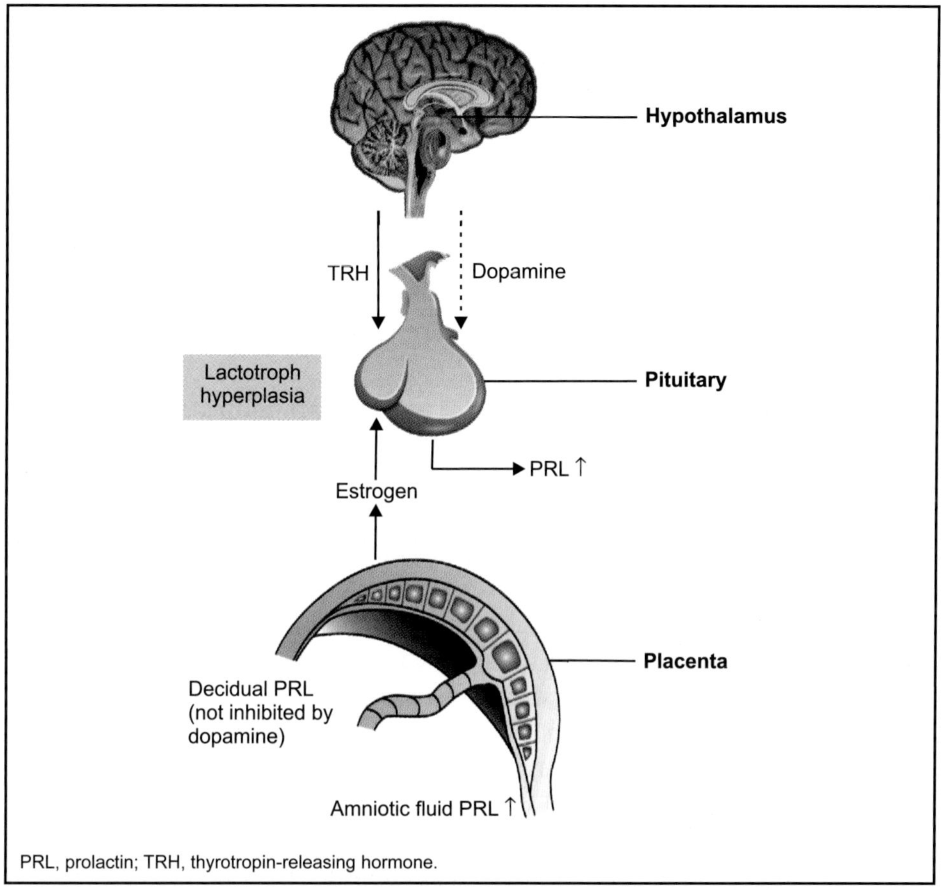

PRL, prolactin; TRH, thyrotropin-releasing hormone.

Figure 1-1 Effect on prolactin secretion by increased estrogen secretion during pregnancy.

Maternal serum concentration of insulin-like growth factor-1 (IGF-1) is elevated during the second half of pregnancy, probably through the combined effect of placental GH-V and HPL. Although the placenta synthesizes and secretes biologically active GnRH, pituitary gonadotropin production decreases during pregnancy.[10] Mean TSH concentrations during the first trimester are significantly lower than in the second and third trimesters or in the nonpregnant state.[18] Most of this early decrease may be due to the intrinsic thyrotropic activity of hCG. A reduction in serum levels of LH and follicle-stimulating hormone (FSH) is also seen. During pregnancy, maternal ACTH levels rise fourfold over concentration in the nonpregnant state between 7 and 10 weeks of gestation. There is a further gradual rise till 33–37 weeks, when a mean fivefold increase over prepregnancy values is found, followed by a 50% drop just before parturition and a marked fifteenfold increase during the stress of delivery.[19] The ACTH concentration returns to the prepregnancy levels within 24 hours of delivery.

Arginine vasopressin (AVP) or antidiuretic hormone (ADH) concentrations in the maternal serum are similar to those in nonpregnant women.[20] Oxytocin levels progressively increase in the maternal blood and parallels the increase in maternal serum estradiol and progesterone. The levels increase further with cervical dilation and vaginal distension during labor and delivery, stimulating contraction of the uterine smooth muscles and enhancing fetal ejection.[21] Uterine oxytocin receptors also increase throughout pregnancy, resulting in a hundredfold increase in oxytocin binding at term in the myometrium.[22]

THYROID GLAND

Evidence of fetal thyroid gland development is apparent early during gestation. Thyroglobulin synthesis can be detected by 4–6 weeks, iodine trapping by 8–10 weeks, and thyroxine (T_4) and, to a lesser extent, triiodothyronine (T_3) synthesis by 12 weeks. Hypothalamic TRH synthesis can be demonstrated by 6–8 weeks and TSH secretion by 12 weeks of gestation. The bilobed-shape of thyroid gland is evident by 7 weeks and thyroid follicles containing colloid by 10 weeks of gestation. There is evidence that transplacental passage of maternal thyroid hormones play an important role in fetal brain development in the first trimester.[23] In light of increased renal clearance of iodine, the status of maternal iodine levels become vital for the development of fetus, as iodine is an essential component for the synthesis of thyroid hormones. The growth and development of the fetus, neurodevelopment in particular, is essentially related to maintenance of maternal euthyroid state. In the first trimester, the fetus relies solely on thyroid hormones and iodine from the mother. Even subtle changes in the thyroid function of the pregnant and lactating woman can cause detrimental effects on the fetus.[24] Fetal T_4 production gradually rises from mid-gestation to term.[25] Fetal serum T_3 levels are relatively lower, owing to placental type 3 deiodinase activity, which converts T_4 to reverse T_3. Maturation of the hypothalamic-pituitary-thyroid axis feedback relationships occurs during the second half of gestation, but it is not complete until after birth. Immediately after birth, there is a TSH surge to 60–80 mIU/L, likely a result of the stress of delivery and clamping of the cord.[26]

The thyroid gland enlarges by an average of 18% during pregnancy. Important changes in thyroidal economy occur due to 3 modifications in the regulation of thyroid hormones. Firstly, pregnancy induces a marked increase in circulating levels of thyroxine-binding globulin (TBG) in response to increasingly high estrogen levels. Secondly, several factors, which have a stimulatory effect on thyroid gland are produced in excess. Lastly, pregnancy is accompanied by a decreased availability of iodine for the maternal thyroid. This occurs because of increased renal clearance and excretion that results in a relative iodine-deficiency state. Thus, there is a twofold increase in TBG and increased total T_4 and T_3 levels in maternal serum throughout pregnancy, whereas for most of the gestation, free T_4 and free T_3 concentrations remain normal.[18]

PARATHYROID GLANDS

During pregnancy, approximately 30 g of calcium is transferred from the maternal compartment to the fetus, with most of the transfer occurring during the last trimester. Maternal total serum calcium levels decrease during pregnancy, with a nadir at 28–32 weeks. This phenomenon is related to the decrease in albumin levels that accompanies the increase in vascular volume.[27] Parathyroid hormone (PTH) plasma concentrations decrease during the first trimester and then increase progressively throughout the remaining pregnancy.[28] Increased levels likely result from the lower calcium concentration in the pregnant woman. Pregnancy and lactation cause profound calcium stress, and during these times, calcitonin levels are appreciably higher than in nonpregnant women. The net result of these actions is a physiological hyperparathyroidism of pregnancy in order to supply the fetus with adequate calcium. The serum levels of 25-hydroxy vitamin D [25(OH)D] are unchanged during pregnancy, but the estrogen-induced rise in vitamin D–binding globulin results in a twofold increase in 1, 25-dihydroxy vitamin D3 [$1,25(OH)_2D3$] concentrations in maternal serum.[27]

ADRENAL GLANDS

During fetal life, there is a remarkable increase in the size of the adrenal glands mainly due to the presence of a well-developed inner zone that involutes after birth.[29] The fetal adrenals are disproportionately large and are larger than the fetal kidneys at mid-gestation.[2] This inner zone comprises 80% of the fetal adrenal cortex at term.[29] The adrenals are as large as those of adults, weighing 10 g or more at term.[2] There is a convincing evidence that the fetal adrenal cortex synthesizes a considerable part of the precursors for estrogen, which are eliminated in the maternal urine during pregnancy. The fetal adrenal glands secrete large quantities of steroid hormones (up to 200 mg daily) near term, and the rate of steroidogenesis is, thus, 5 times of that observed in the adrenal glands of resting adults. Also, the fetal adrenal cortex is one of the main users of placental progesterone in its synthesis of adrenocortical hormones.[29]As clinically evidenced, ACTH is the primary trophic hormone of the fetal adrenal glands. ACTH-related peptides, growth factors, and other hormones have been suggested as possible contributory trophic hormones for the fetal zone. The adrenal glands shrink to almost 50% in size, because of regression of fetal zonal cells after birth.[2]

In normal pregnancy, the maternal adrenal glands undergo little, if any, morphological change.[3] As a result of the hyperestrogenemia of pregnancy, hepatic production of cortisol-binding globulin is increased. The increased production results in doubling of the maternal serum levels of cortisol-binding globulin, which in turn results in decreased metabolic clearance of cortisol and a threefold rise in total plasma cortisol by 26 weeks, when the levels reach a plateau until they rise at the onset of labor. The enhanced cortisol production is due to an increase in the maternal plasma ACTH concentrations and hyperresponsiveness of the adrenal cortex to ACTH stimulation during pregnancy.[19] Cortisol secretion follows that of ACTH, and the diurnal rhythm is maintained during pregnancy. Despite the elevated free cortisol levels, pregnant women do not develop the stigma of glucocorticoid excess, possibly because of the antiglucocorticoid activities of the elevated concentrations of progesterone.[30]

As early as 15 weeks, the maternal adrenal glands secrete considerably increased amounts of aldosterone. By the third trimester, about 1 mg/day is secreted. If sodium intake is restricted, aldosterone secretion is elevated even further.[31] At the same time, levels of renin and angiotensin II substrate normally are increased, especially during the latter half of pregnancy. This scenario gives rise to increased plasma levels of angiotensin II, which by acting on the zona glomerulosa of the maternal adrenal glands, accounts for the markedly elevated aldosterone secretion. It has been suggested that the increased aldosterone secretion during normal pregnancy affords protection against the natriuretic effect of progesterone and atrial natriuretic peptide.

Maternal plasma androstenedione and testosterone are increased in pregnancy. These hormones are converted to estradiol in placenta, which increases their clearance rates. Conversely, the increased sex hormone-binding globulin (SHBG) in plasma of pregnant women retards testosterone clearance.[3]

Adrenal medullary function remains normal throughout pregnancy. Thus, 24-hour urine catecholamine and plasma epinephrine and norepinephrine levels are similar to concentrations in the nonpregnant state.[32]

PANCREAS

Hyperplasia and hypertrophy of β cells in the islets of Langerhans are probably the result of stimulation by estrogen and progesterone.[33] During early pregnancy, the glucose requirement of the fetus leads to enhanced transport of glucose across the placenta by facilitated diffusion, and maternal fasting hypoglycemia may be present. Although basal insulin levels may be normal, there is hypersecretion of insulin in response to a meal. Because the half-life of insulin is not altered during pregnancy,[34] this increase represents an increase in synthesis and secretion. This results in enhanced glycogen storage and decreased hepatic glucose production.

As pregnancy progresses, the levels of HPL rise, as do the levels of glucocorticoids, leading to insulin resistance (IR) found during the last half of pregnancy.[35] Thus, in late pregnancy, glucose ingestion results in higher and more sustained levels of glucose and insulin and a greater degree of glucagon suppression than in the nonpregnant state.

CONCLUSION

The maternal endocrinological activities and processes play a vital as well as critical role in the initiation and maintenance of pregnancy. The interplay of these processes is essential in the complete period of pregnancy and the requirements of the fetus, even after birth. Progesterone and estrogen are primarily concerned with the maintenance of the gestational period and preparing the mother for further requirements and necessities of the fetus. While hCG is responsible for the continued progesterone production during gestation, HPL ensures fetal nutrition and angiogenesis. Thyroid hormones are responsible for the growth and development, especially neurodevelopment of the fetus, and hyperparathyroidism ensures adequate availability of calcium to the fetus. ACTH ensures the maintenance of the diurnal rhythm during pregnancy, and aldosterone provides protection against natriuretic effect of the progesterone and atrial natriuretic peptide. All the maternal hormones, thus, synchronize with each other and result in the evolution of a new life.

REFERENCES

1. King JC. Physiology of pregnancy and nutrient metabolism. *Am J Clin Nutr*. 2000;71: 1218S-25S.
2. Feldt–Rasmussen U, Mathiesen ER. Endocrine disorders in pregnancy: Physiological and hormonal aspects of pregnancy. *Best Pract Res Clin Endocrinol Metab*. 2011;25:875-84.
3. Maternal Physiology. In: Cunningham FG, Leveno KJ, Bloom SL, Hauth JC, Gilstrap LC III, Wenstrom KD eds. Williams Obstetrics. 22nd edition. New York: McGraw-Hill Publications; 2007.
4. Braunstein GD. Endocrine changes in pregnancy. In: Melmed S, Polonsky KS, Larsen PR, Kronenberg HM eds. Williams Textbook of Endocrinology. 12th edition. Mosby:Saunders Elsevier; 2011. p. 819-33.
5. Diczfalusy E, Troen P. Endocrine functions of the human placenta. *Vitams Horm*. 1961; 19:229.
6. Pepe GJ, Albrecht ED. Actions of placental and fetal adrenal steroid hormones in primate pregnancy. *Endocr Rev*. 1995;16:608-48.
7. McGregor WG, Kuhn RW, Jaffe RB. Biologically active chorionic gonadotropin: synthesis by the human fetus. *Science*. 1983;220:306.
8. Handwerger S, Brar A. Placental lactogen, placental growth hormone, and decidual prolactin. *Seminars Reprod Endocrinol*. 1992;10:106.
9. Corbacho AM, Martinez De La Escalere G, Clapp C. Roles of prolactin and related members of the prolactin/growth hormone/placental lactogen family in angiogenesis. *J Endocrinol*. 2002;173:219-38.
10. Foyouzi N, Frisbaek Y, Norwitz ER. Pituitary gland and pregnancy. *Obstet Gynecol Clin North Am*. 2004;31:873-92.
11. Elster AD, Sanders TG, Vines FS, Chen MY. Size and shape of the pituitary gland during pregnancy and post-partum: measurement with MR imaging. *Radiology*. 1991;181:531-5.

12. Lehtovirta P, Ranta T. Effect of short-term bromocriptine treatment on amniotic fluid prolactin concentration in the first half of pregnancy. *Acta Endocrinol (Copenh).* 1981;97: 559-61.
13. Andersen JR. Prolactin in amniotic fluid and maternal serum during uncomplicated human pregnancy. *Dan Med Bull.* 1982;29:266-74.
14. Emmi AM, Skurnick J, Goldsmith LT, Gagliardi CL, Schmidt CL, Kleinberg D, et al. Ovarian control of pituitary hormone secretion in early human pregnancy. *J Clin Endocrinol Metab.* 1991;72:1359-63.
15. Kletzky OA, Rossman F, Bertolli SI, Platt LD, Mishell DR Jr. Dynamics of human chorionic gonadotropin, prolactin, and growth hormone in serum and amniotic fluid throughout normal human pregnancy. *Am J Obstet Gynecol.* 1985;151:878-84.
16. Lønberg U, Damm P, Andersson AM, Maink M, Chellakooty M, Laurenborg J, et al. Increase in maternal placental growth hormone during pregnancy and disappearance during parturition in normal and growth hormone-deficient pregnancies. *Am J Obstet Gynecol.* 2003;188:247-51.
17. Obuobie K, Mullik V, Jones C, John R, Rees AE, Davies JS, et al. McCune-Albright syndrome: Growth hormone dynamics in pregnancy. *J Clin Endocrinol Metab.* 2001;86:2456-8.
18. Glinoer D. The regulation of thyroid function in pregnancy: pathways of endocrine adaptation from physiology to pathology. *Endocr Rev.* 1997;18:404-33.
19. Lindsay JR, Nieman LK. The hypothalamic-pituitary-adrenal axis in pregnancy: challenges in disease detection and treatment. *Endocrin Rev.* 2005;26:775-99.
20. Davison JM, Shiells EA, Philips PR, Lindheimer MD. Serial evaluation of vasopressin release and thirst in human pregnancy. Role of human chorionic gonadotrophin in the osmoregulatory changes of gestation. *J Clin Invest.* 1988;81:798-806.
21. Leake RD, Weitzman RE, Glatz TH, Fisher DA. Plasma oxytocin concentrations in men, nonpregnant women, and pregnant women before and during spontaneous labor. *J Clin Endocrinol Metab.* 1981;53:730-3.
22. Zeeman GG, Khan-Dawood FS, Dawood MY. Oxytocin and its receptor in pregnancy and parturition: current concepts and clinical implications. *Obstet Gynecol.* 1997;89: 873-83.
23. Raymond J, LaFranchi SH. Fetal and neonatal thyroid function: review and summary of significant new findings. *Curr Opin Endocrinol Diabetes Obes.* 2010;17:1-7.
24. Henrichs J, Bongers-Schokking JJ, Schenk JJ, Ghassabian A, Schmidt HG, Visser TJ, et al. Maternal thyroid function during early pregnancy and cognitive functioning in early childhood: the generation R study. *J Clin Endocrinol Metab.* 2010;95:4227-34.
25. Thorpe-Beeston JG, Nicolaides KH, Felton CV, Butler J, McGregor AM. Maturation of the secretion of thyroid hormone and thyroid-stimulating hormone in the fetus. *N Engl J Med.* 1991;324:532-6.
26. Brown RS, Huang SA, Fisher DA. The maturation of thyroid function in the perinatal period and during childhood. In: Braverman LE, Utiger RD, eds. Werner's and Ingbar's the thyroid. Philadelphia, Pennsylvania: Lippincott Williams and Wilkins; 2000. pp. 1013-28.
27. Kovacs CS. Calcium and bone metabolism in pregnancy and lactation. *J Clin Endocrinol Metab.* 2001;86:2344-8.
28. Pitkin RM, Reynolds WA, Williams GA, Hargis GK. Calcium metabolism in normal pregnancy: A longitudinal study. *Am J Obstet Gynecol.* 1979;133:781-90.

29. Johannison E. The foetal adrenal cortex in the human. *Acta Endocrinol (Copenh)*. 1968;58:7.
30. Carr BR, Parker CR Jr, Madden JD, MacDonald PC, Porter JC. Maternal plasma adrenocorticotropin and cortisol relationships throughout human pregnancy. *Am J Obstet Gynecol*. 1981;139:416-22.
31. Watanabe M, Meeker CI, Gray MJ, Sims EA, Solomon S. Secretion rate of aldosterone in normal pregnancy. *J Clin Invest*. 1963;42:1619-31.
32. Zuspan FP. Urinary excretion of epinephrine and norepinephrine during pregnancy. *J Clin Endocrinol Metab*. 1970;30:357-60.
33. Costrini NV, Kalkhoff RK. Relative effects of pregnancy, estradiol, and progesterone on plasma insulin and pancreatic islet insulin secretion. *J Clin Invest*. 1971;50:992-9.
34. Lind T, Bell S, Gilmore E, Huisjes HJ, Schally AV. Insulin disappearance rate in pregnant and non-pregnant women, and in non-pregnant women given GHRIH. *Eur J Clin Invest*. 1977;7:47-52.
35. Galerneau F, Inzucchi SE. Diabetes mellitus in pregnancy. *Obstet Gynecol Clin North Am*. 2004;31:907-33.

2

Pregnancy and Diabetes Mellitus

Rajesh Rajput

INTRODUCTION

Pregnancy may be complicated by diabetes in two ways: pregestational diabetes and gestational diabetes. Diabetes that antedates pregnancy is called pregestational diabetes while the one that develops for the first time during pregnancy is called gestational diabetes.

PREGESTATIONAL DIABETES

Pregnancy complicated by preexisting type 1 or type 2 diabetes mellitus poses additional risk to both mother and fetus. Uncontrolled hyperglycemia present at the time of conception and, thereafter, during first trimester (critical period for fetal organogenesis), increases the chances of spontaneous abortion and risk of congenital malformations in the developing fetus (Table 2-1).[1]

The incidence of congenital malformations in fetuses is 5–9% in women with uncontrolled diabetes as compared to 2% in general population. Since malformations

TABLE 2-1

Risk of Congenital Malformations in Infants of Diabetic Mother	
• Caudal regression	• Anencephaly
• Spina bifida, hydrocephalus and other caudal NTDs	• Anal/rectal atresia
• Cardiac anomalies	• Renal anomalies
– Transposition of great vessel	– Agenesis
– Ventricular septal defect	– Cystic kidney
– Atrial septal defect	– Ureter duplex
	• Situs inversus

NTDs, neural tube defects.

commonly associated with diabetes occur before 7th week of gestation, the intervention to control hyperglycemia and reduce the risk of malformations must begin before conception.[1,2] The preconception goals are described in table 2-2.[3]

The presence of complications like retinopathy, neuropathy, nephropathy, hypertension, hypercholesterolemia, and hypoglycemic unawareness developed secondary to uncontrolled diabetes prior to conception poses additional risk. Thus, in all diabetic women becoming pregnant, risk stratification should be done using White classification of diabetes during pregnancy (Table 2-3).[4]

Various studies have demonstrated very little difference in outcome in classes B, C, and D whereas class F diabetes increases the risk of maternal hypertensive

TABLE 2-2

Preconception Target of Blood Glucose in Diabetic Women

Goal	*Plasma glucose (mg/dL)*	*Whole blood glucose (mg/dL)*
Fasting and premeal glucose	80–110	70–100
2-hour postprandial	100–155	90–140
HbA1c	<7%; as close to normal as possible without subjecting the women to risk of hypoglycemia	

HbA1c, glycosylated hemoglobin.

Source: American Diabetes Association. Preconception care of women with diabetes. *Diabetes Care.* 2004;27:S76-S8.

TABLE 2-3

White Classification (Revised) of Diabetes During Pregnancy

Gestational diabetes	Abnormal glucose tolerance, but euglycemia maintained by diet alone or if diet alone insufficient, insulin required
Class A	Diet alone sufficient, any duration or age of onset
Class B	Age of onset ≥20 years and duration <10 years
Class C	Age of onset 10–19 years and duration 10–19 years
Class D	Age of onset <10 years and duration ≥20 years or background retinopathy or hypertension (not preeclampsia)
Class R	Proliferative retinopathy or vitreous hemorrhage
Class F	Nephropathy with proteinuria >500 mg/dL
Class RF	Criteria for both classes R and F coexist
Class H	Arteriosclerotic heart diseases clinically evident
Class T	Prior renal transplantation

Source: Hare J, White P. Gestational diabetes and the White classification. *Diabetes Care.* 1980;3:394.

complications and fetal intrauterine growth retardation (IUGR) and prematurity. Presence of microalbuminuria alone increases the risk for preeclampsia by 30% while presence of both hypertension and microalbuminuria increases the risk by 50%. A lower case "f" could be used to distinguish this additional risk in classes B, C, D, and R.

GESTATIONAL DIABETES MELLITUS

Gestational diabetes mellitus (GDM) is defined as glucose intolerance that begins or is first detected during pregnancy irrespective of treatment with diet or insulin. Depending on the population sample and diagnostic criteria, the prevalence may range from 1 to 14% of all pregnancies complicated by diabetes.[5]

Pathophysiology

The metabolic goals of pregnancy are to develop anabolic stores in early pregnancy in order to meet metabolic demands for fetal growth and energy in late pregnancy. This fine tuning of glycemic levels during pregnancy is possibly due to the compensatory hyperinsulinemia, as the normal pregnancy is characterized by insulin resistance (IR). IR usually begins in the second trimester and progresses throughout the remaining pregnancy. Insulin sensitivity is reduced by as much as 80%. Placental secretion of hormones, such as progesterone, cortisol, human placental lactogen (HPL), and growth hormone is a major contributor to the insulin-resistant state seen in pregnancy. The IR likely plays a role in ensuring that the fetus has an adequate supply of glucose by changing the maternal energy metabolism from carbohydrates to lipids. A pregnant woman who is not able to increase her insulin secretion to overcome the IR that occurs during normal pregnancy also develops gestational diabetes.[6]

Screening

There is no worldwide agreement on the best way to screen for GDM. Previously, universal screening at 24–28 weeks of gestation with a 50 g oral glucose challenge test was recommended. However, based on results of various studies, American Diabetes Association (ADA)[7] now recommends selective screening depending upon risk stratification of pregnant women (Table 2-4). Women with a 1 hour glucose level of more than 140 mg/dL were referred for a diagnostic oral glucose tolerance test (OGTT). This test can be done at any time of the day when pregnant women visit their consulting physician, irrespective of the last meal.

If a woman is at high risk, glucose testing should be done as soon as possible. If the initial testing is negative, the woman should be retested between 24 and 28 weeks of gestation. If she is at intermediate risk, she should undergo glucose testing at 24–28 weeks. If she is at low risk, the ADA does not recommend screening for GDM.

TABLE 2-4

Risk Stratification of Pregnant Women		
High risk for GDM	*Intermediate risk for GDM*	*Low risk for GDM*
• Marked obesity • Personal history of GDM, glucose intolerance, or glycosuria • A strong family history of type 2 diabetes • History of PCOS.	• A woman is considered to be at intermediate risk if she does not fit into either the high- or low-risk category.	• Age <25 years • Normal pregnancy weight • Not a member of an ethnic/racial group with a high prevalence of diabetes (e.g., Hispanic American, Native American, Asian American, African American, or Pacific Islander) • No known diabetes in first-degree relatives • No history of abnormal glucose tolerance and no history of poor obstetric outcome.

GDM, gestational diabetes mellitus; PCOS, polycystic ovary syndrome.

Source: American Diabetes Association. Standards of medical care in diabetes—2007. *Diabetes Care.* 2007;30:S4-S41.

There are 2 approaches for screening of GDM. Women at low risk are subjected to 50 g oral glucose challenge test and if positive, they are further subjected to OGTT. The high risk women are subjected to OGTT directly without prior screening with 50-g 1 hour glucose challenge test and is called 'one-step approach'. Since Indian women have elevenfold higher risk of developing dysglycemia during pregnancy, one step approach should be followed.

Diagnostic Criteria

OGTT is used for detection and diagnosis of GDM. It is performed after an overnight fast of at least 8 hours and not more than 14 hours and after at least 3 days of unrestricted diet, including carbohydrate intake of more than 150 g per day. Patient needs to remain seated and should not smoke during the test. OGTT most commonly used to diagnose GDM in the US is a 3-hour 100 g OGTT. According to diagnostic criteria recommended by the ADA,[7] GDM is diagnosed if 2 or more plasma glucose levels meet or exceed the following thresholds:

- Fasting glucose concentration of 95 mg/dL
- 1 hour glucose concentration of 180 mg/dL
- 2-hour glucose concentration of 155 mg/dL, or
- 3-hour glucose concentration of 140 mg/dL.

ADA recommendations also include the use of a 2-hour 75 g OGTT with the same glucose thresholds listed for fasting, 1 hour, and 2-hour values. The World Health Organization (WHO)[8] diagnostic criteria, which is used in many countries outside North America, is based on a 2-hour 75 g OGTT. GDM is diagnosed by WHO criteria if either the fasting glucose is more than 126 mg/dL or the 2-hour glucose is more than 140 mg/dL. More recently, International Association of Diabetes and Pregnancy Study Group (IADPSG),[9] based on findings of Hyperglycemia and Adverse Pregnancy Outcome (HAPO)[10] study recommended that GDM should be diagnosed if one or more plasma glucose values equaled or exceeded the recommended threshold. The Diabetes in Pregnancy Study Group India (DIPSI)[11] gave their own recommendations which were similar to WHO recommendations. Table 2-5 summarizes various criteria used for the diagnosis of GDM.

Which Criteria to Use?

The Brazilian Gestational Diabetes Study[12] evaluated the ADA and WHO diagnostic criteria against pregnancy outcomes in an observational cohort. Both the criteria predicted an increased risk of macrosomia, preeclampsia, and perinatal death. The study concluded that both ADA and WHO criteria can be used as valid options in establishing the diagnosis of GDM and predicting the adverse outcomes during pregnancy. Given the complexities of different cutoffs given by various guidelines and uncertainties surrounding them, it is recommended to use ADA criteria till the time more data are made available documenting the clear superiority of one over the other.

Management

Appropriate management of diabetes involves proper dietary advice, oral drugs, and insulin therapy either alone or in combination. There is no one fit therapy for all women

TABLE 2-5

Various Diagnostic Criteria for GDM

Diagnostic criteria for GDM	*ADA 100 g OGTT*	*ADA 75 g OGTT*	*WHO 75 g OGTT*	*HAPO 75 g OGTT*	*DIPSI*
FPG (mg/dL)	95	95	126	92	–
1 hour plasma glucose (mg/dL)	180	180	–	180	–
2-hour plasma glucose (mg/dL)	155	155	140	153	>140
3-hour plasma glucose (mg/dL)	140	–	–	–	–

GDM, gestational diabetes mellitus; ADA, American Diabetes Association; WHO, World Health Organization; HAPO, Hyperglycemia and Adverse Pregnancy Outcome; DIPSI, Diabetes in Pregnancy Study Group India; OGTT, oral glucose tolerance test; FPG, fasting plasma glucose.

TABLE 2-6

Post-conception Goals of Blood Glucose Levels		
Goal	*Plasma glucose (mg/dL)*	*Whole blood glucose (mg/dL)*
Fasting and premeal glucose	70–105	60–95
1-hour postprandial glucose	100–155	90–140
2-hour postprandial glucose	90–130	80–120

Source: American Diabetes Association. Gestational Diabetes Mellitus. *Diabetes Care.* 2003;27:S88-S90.

and treatment needs to be individualized. During pregnancy, normal fasting plasma glucose level is around 89 mg/dL and 2 hours plasma glucose level is 122 mg/dL; a mean plasma glucose (MPG) value of 105–110 mg/dL is desirable for a good maternal and fetal outcome. The postconception goals are given in table 2-6.[13]

Medical Nutrition Therapy

The goals of medical nutrition therapy (MNT) are to provide adequate nutrition for the mother and fetus, provide sufficient calories for appropriate maternal weight gain, maintain normoglycemia, and avoid ketosis. In general, an increased energy requirement is not present during the first trimester of pregnancy. However, most normal weight women require an additional 300 kcal/day in the second and third trimesters. In normal weight women with GDM, the recommended daily caloric intake is 30 kcal/kg/day based on their present pregnancy weight. In women with GDM who are overweight [having weight 120–150% of ideal body weight (body mass index—BMI >30 kg/m^2)], a 33% calorie restriction, i.e., 25 kcal/kg/day is recommended; while in those women having less than 80% ideal body weight, a calorie intake of 40 kcal/kg/day based on their present pregnancy weight is recommended. It is suggested to avoid intake of a single large meal and foods with a large percentage of simple carbohydrates. A total of 6 feedings per day is preferred, with 3 major meals and 3 snacks to limit the degree of glycemic excursion in view of compromised β-cell reserve. The diet should include foods with complex carbohydrates and cellulose, such as whole grain breads and legumes. Carbohydrates should not account for more than 50% of the calories, with protein and fats equally accounting for the remainder.[14,15]

Unless contraindicated, all pregnant women with diabetes should be encouraged to do some degree of exercise. The appropriate diet and exercise leads to significant decrease in both fasting and postprandial plasma glucose levels as compared to diet alone. During exercise, women are advised to palpate their uterus to detect subclinical uterine contractions and to discontinue the exercise if contractions occur. Uterine activity, defined as contractions with an external tocometer deflection of more than 15 mmHg above baseline for more than 30 seconds varies in response to different types of aerobic exercise, even at comparable levels of exertion. The bicycle ergometer, treadmill, and rowing ergometer lead to uterine activity in 50%, 40%, and 10% of exercise sessions, respectively. The recumbent bicycle and upper body ergometer do not lead to any increase in uterine activity. Therefore, it is recommended that the recumbent bicycle and upper body ergometer are the safest forms of aerobic exercise for pregnant women. Absolute contraindications to exercise during pregnancy include preterm labor, premature rupture of membranes (PROM), incompetent cervix, persistent second and or third trimester bleeding, IUGR, placenta previa beyond 26 weeks, and pregnancy induced hypertension.[16,17]

Oral Agents

Currently, oral hypoglycemic agents are not recommended by the ADA or American Congress of Obstetricians and Gynecologist (ACOG). However, 2 oral drugs, glibenclamide and metformin are used during pregnancy, and trials have found these agents to be safe and effective, although the potential for long-term adverse effects remains a concern. The transfer of glibenclamide, a second-generation sulfonylurea, across the human placenta was insignificant in experimental models. This finding led to a clinical trial of 404 women with GDM randomized to either glibenclamide or insulin therapy at 11–33 weeks of gestation. There were no significant differences in glycemic control or adverse fetal outcomes. In addition, glibenclamide was not detected in the cord serum of any infant in the glibenclamide group.[18] However, till date, glibenclamide is considered to be in Pregnancy Category C by the US Food and Drug Administration (FDA) and, therefore, it is not currently recommended by the ADA or ACOG until larger studies confirm its safety. Success rates for achieving glycemic control with glibenclamide vary from 79 to 86%. Studies evaluating predictors of failure with glibenclamide involves the following risk factors: advanced maternal age, earlier gestational age at diagnosis, higher gravidity and parity, and higher mean fasting glucose level.[19] If used, the woman should not be in the first trimester, because its effects, if any, on the embryo are unknown. It has been shown to be safe in breastfeeding, as it is not excreted in human milk.

Metformin has also been used to treat pregnant women with GDM. Various studies involving women with PCOS or women with type 2 diabetes mellitus who continue metformin during pregnancy, have no adverse pregnancy outcomes. Metformin is considered as Category B by the FDA during pregnancy.[20,21]

Insulin

Insulin therapy is most commonly used when MNT fails to maintain blood plasma glucose levels at the desired ranges, i.e., fasting plasma glucose below 105 mg/dL, 1 hour postprandial plasma glucose below 155 mg/dL and 2-hour postprandial plasma glucose below 130 mg/dL, or when there is an evidence of excessive fetal growth. Various studies have demonstrated a decrease in the incidence of macrosomia, cesarean section, fetal metabolic complications, shoulder dystocia, neonatal intensive care unit days, and respiratory complications in women with GDM who were treated with insulin. The average insulin requirement during pregnancy is 0.7 IU/kg/day but it needs to be individualized as IR increases from 20 weeks of gestation onwards till 32 weeks, when it stabilizes. The optimal insulin regimen should include the type and dose of insulin tailored to meet each patient's requirements. Insulins lispro, aspart, regular and neutral protamine hagedorn (NPH) are well studied in pregnancy and are regarded as safe and effective and are currently recommended by the ADA. Long-acting insulin analogues, i.e., glargine and levemir are less well-studied, but are used successfully during pregnancy. When more than 20% of postprandial blood glucose levels exceed 130 mg/dL, short-acting insulin analogue, i.e., aspart or insulin in dosage of 4–8 IU subcutaneously (SC) should be given before meals. If more than 10 U of short acting insulin is needed before the noon meal, adding 8–12 IU of NPH insulin before breakfast helps achieve control. When more than 10% of fasting glucose levels exceeds 95 mg/dL, initiate 6–8 IU NPH insulin at bedtime. Dosage of insulin should be titrated to maintain plasma glucose in target range as well as to avoid hypoglycemia.[22-24]

Insulin Pump

In a selected group of patients, use of an insulin pump may improve glycemic control while enhancing patient convenience. These devices can be programmed to infuse varying basal and bolus levels of insulin, which change smoothly even while the patient sleeps or is otherwise preoccupied. The cannula used to infuse insulin needs to be changed after 3 days.[25]

Role of Glucose Monitoring

Self monitoring of blood glucose is recommended for women with GDM. The goal of monitoring is to detect glucose concentrations elevated enough to increase perinatal mortality. It should be performed a minimum of 4 times a day, including before breakfast and 2 hours after the 3 major meals. It is important to check postprandial glucose levels, because these have been shown to correlate more with the macrosomia than the fasting levels. In women with GDM who require insulin therapy, adjustments in the incidence of therapy should be based on postprandial, rather than preprandial glucose levels. One prospective study of 668 patients (334 with GDM and 334 control subjects) found that women with GDM who had a mean blood glucose level between 87 and 104 mg/dL had incidence rates of IUGR and large for gestational age (LGA) infants comparable to the control group. However, women who had mean blood glucose values below 87 mg/dL had a higher incidence of infants with IUGR, whereas women who had mean blood glucose values above 104 mg/dL had a higher incidence of LGA infants. This study suggests that although it is important to treat hyperglycemia in GDM, it is also important not to over treat because this can increase the risk of IUGR.[26]

Labor and Delivery

Timing of delivery should be selected to minimize morbidity for the mother and the fetus. It should be carried out as near as possible to the expected date, as it helps to maximize cervical maturity and improves the chances of spontaneous labor and vaginal delivery. Euglycemia should be maintained during labor or prior to a scheduled cesarean section. The method of delivery depends on fetal weight. Cesarean section should be recommended for fetus weighing more than 4.5 kg; however, these guidelines may be individualized based on prior obstetric history and adequacy of pelvic size. Patients should be instructed to take their usual bedtime dose of insulin the night prior to delivery. On the day of delivery, intermediate/long acting insulin can be withheld and either glucose insulin potassium drip (GIK) or separate intravenous insulin drip and 5% dextrose should be started to maintain blood glucose in the target range of 80–110 mg/dL. In case of prolonged labor, 5% dextrose should be administered at a rate of 100 mL/hour to avoid starvation ketosis. In pregnant women with preeclampsia, 10% dextrose at rate of 50 mL/hour should be used to avoid fluid overload. One should avoid giving boluses of dextrose to the mother during delivery, except when needed to correct severe hypoglycemia as elevated maternal blood glucose levels increase the risk of neonatal hypoglycemia, hypoxia, and acidosis.[27,28]

Postpartum Management

After delivery of placenta, IR decreases markedly and thus, to avoid hypoglycemia, the insulin dosage should be reduced by half during first 24 hours after the delivery. By 2 weeks postpartum, insulin requirement stabilizes, and its dosage should be adjusted accordingly. The woman should be reassessed at 6 weeks postpartum for microalbuminuria, glycosylated hemoglobin (HbA1c), and fundus examination. The American Academy of Pediatrics (AAP) considers angiotensin converting enzyme inhibitors (ACEi) safe for use by breastfeeding mothers and it should be restarted in patients with nephropathy, microalbuminuria, and hypertension.[29] Importance of contraception should be discussed at this point of time as, all diabetic women must delay future pregnancies until they are medically stable and have achieved near euglycemia. If oral contraceptive pills are chosen as method of contraception, combined estrogen-progesterone pills are preferred over progesterone only pills as the latter have been found to be associated with increased risk of development of type 2 diabetes.[30]

In most cases of GDM, glucose intolerance resolves after delivery of placenta and neither insulin nor drugs are needed. However, earlier the glucose intolerance develops in pregnancy and the more extreme the insulin requirement is, the condition is less likely to resolve completely in the postpartum period. In those women where glucose levels remain elevated, insulin therapy is indicated, as most oral agents are excreted in breast milk. GDM recurs approximately in 50% of subsequent pregnancies. The future risk of developing diabetes for a gestational diabetic is twofold, if she becomes overweight and, therefore, gestational diabetic women require follow-up. Glucose tolerance test with 75 g oral glucose is performed after 6 weeks of delivery, and if necessary, is repeated after 6 months and every year to determine whether the glucose tolerance has returned to normal or progressed.[31]

CONCLUSION

Diabetes mellitus, whether gestational or pregestational, is found to be associated with multiple maternal and fetal complications. It can also result in congenital malformations in the fetus. Prompt screening, diagnosis, and apt therapeutic as well as lifestyle modifications can help in greatly reducing the complications and lead to a normal pregnancy and delivery of healthy infant.

REFERENCES

1. Mills JL, Baker L, Goldman AS. Malformations in infants of diabetic mothers occur before seventh gestational week. Implications for treatment. *Diabetes*. 1979;28:292-3.
2. Kitzmiller JL, Buchanan TA, Kjos S, Coombs AC, Ratner RE. Pre-conception care of diabetes, congenital malformations, and spontaneous abortions. *Diabetes Care*. 1996;19: 514-41.
3. American Diabetes Association. Preconception care of women with diabetes. *Diabetes Care*. 2004;27:S76-S8.
4. Hare JW, White P. Gestational diabetes and the White classification. *Diabetes Care*. 1980; 3:394.
5. Ben-Haroush A, Yogev Y, Hod M. Epidemiology of gestational diabetes mellitus and its association with Type 2 diabetes. *Diabet Med*. 2004;21:103-13.
6. Di Cianni GD, Miccoli R, Volpe L, Lencioni C, Del Prato S. Intermediate metabolism in normal pregnancy and in gestational diabetes. *Diabetes Metab Res Rev*. 2003;19:259-70.
7. American Diabetes Association. Standards of medical care in diabetes—2007. *Diabetes Care*. 2007;30:S4-S41.
8. Setji TL, Brown AJ, Feinglos MN. Gestational diabetes mellitus. *Clinical Diabetes*. 2005; 30:17-24.
9. International Association of Diabetes and Pregnancy Study Groups Consensus Panel, Metzger BE, Gabbe SG, Persson B, Buchanan TA, Catalano PA, et al. International association of diabetes and pregnancy study groups recommendations on the diagnosis and classification of hyperglycemia in pregnancy. *Diabetes Care*. 2010;33:676-82.
10. HAPO Study Cooperative Research Group, Metzger BE, Lowe LP, Dyer AR, Trimble ER, Chaovarindr U, et al. Hyperglycemia and adverse pregnancy outcomes. *N Engl J Med*. 2008;358:1991-2002.
11. Seshiah V, Sahay BK, Das AK, Shah S, Banerjee S, Rao PV, et al. Gestational Diabetes Mellitus – Indian Guidelines. *J Indian Med Assoc*. 2009;107:799-802, 804-6.

12. Schmidt MI, Duncan BB, Reichelt AJ, Branchtein L, Matos MC, Costa e Forti A, et al; Brazillian Gestational Diabetes Study Group. Gestational diabetes mellitus diagnosed with a 2-h 75 g oral glucose tolerance test and adverse pregnancy outcomes. *Diabetes Care.* 2001;24:1151-5.
13. American Diabetes Association. Gestational Diabetes Mellitus. *Diabetes Care.* 2003;27: S88-S90.
14. Franz MJ, Bantle JP, Beebe CA, Brunzell JD, Chiasson JL, Gareg A, et al. Evidence based nutrition principles and recommendations for the treatment and prevention of diabetes and related complications. *Diabetes Care.* 2002;25:148-98.
15. Jovanovic-Peterson L, Peterson CM. Nutritional management of the obese gestational diabetic pregnant women. *J Am Coll Nutr.* 1992;11:246-50.
16. Harris GD. Exercise and the pregnant patient: a clinical overview. *Women Health Primary Care.* 2005;8:79-86.
17. ACOG Committee Obstetric Practice. ACOG committee opinion. Number 267, January 2002: exercise during pregnancy and the postpartum period. *Obstet Gynecol.* 2001;99: 171-3.
18. Langer O, Conway DL, Berkus MD, Xenakis EM, Gonzales O. A comparison of glyburide and insulin in women with gestational diabetes mellitus. *N Engl J Med.* 2000;343:1134-8.
19. Kahn BF, Davies JK, Lynch AM, Reynolds RM, Barbour LA. Predictors of glyburide failure in the treatment of gestational diabetes. *Obstet Gynecol.* 2006;107:1303-9.
20. Glueck CJ, Phillips H, Cameron D, Sieve-Smith L, Wang P. Continuing metformin throughout pregnancy in women with polycystic ovary syndrome appears to safely reduce first-trimester spontaneous abortion: a pilot study. *Fertil Steril.* 2001;75:46-52.
21. Goh JE, Sadler L, Rowan J. Metformin for gestational diabetes in routine clinical practice. *Diabet Med.* 2011;28:1082-7.
22. Thompson DJ, Porter KB, Gunnells DJ, Wagner PC, Spinnato JA. Prophylactic insulin in the management of gestational diabetes. *Obstet Gynecol.* 1990;75:960-4.
23. Coustan DR, Imarah J. Prophylactic insulin treatment of gestational diabetes reduces the incidence of macrosomia, operative delivery, and birth trauma. *Am J Obstet Gynecol.* 1984;150:836-42.
24. Langer O, Rodriguez DA, Xenakis EM, McFarland MB, Berkus MD, Arredondo F. Intensified versus conventional management of gestational diabetes. *Am J Obstet Gynecol.* 1994;170:1036-47.
25. Gabbe SG, Holing E, Temple P, Brown ZA. Benefits, risks, costs, and patient satisfaction associated with insulin pump therapy for the pregnancy complicated by type 1 diabetes mellitus. *Am J Obstet Gynecol.* 2000;182:1283-91.
26. Langer O, Levy J, Brustman L, Anyaegbunam A, Merkatz R, Divon M. Glycemic control in gestational diabetes mellitus: how tight is tight enough: small for gestational age versus large for gestational age? *Am J Obstet Gynecol.* 1989;161:646-53.
27. Naylor CD, Sermer M, Chen E, Sykora K. Cesarean delivery in relation to birth weight and gestational glucose tolerance: pathophysiology or practice style? Toronto tri-hospital gestational diabetes investigators. *JAMA.* 1999;275:1165-70.
28. American College of Obstetrics and Gynecologists Committee on Practice Bulletins-Obstetrics. ACOG Practice Bulletin. Clinical management guidelines for obstetricians-

gynecologists. Number 30, September 2001 (replace Technical Bulletin Number 200, December 1994). Gestational diabetes. *Obstet Gynecol.* 2001;98:525-38.

29. ACOG Committee on Practice Bulletins. ACOG Practice Bulletin. Chronic hypertension in pregnancy. ACOG Committee on Practice Bulletins. *Obstet Gynecol.* 2001;98:177-84.
30. Kjos SL, Peters RK, Xiang A, Thomas D, Schaefer U, Buchanan TA. Contraception and the risk of type 2 diabetes mellitus in Latina women with prior gestational diabetes mellitus. *JAMA*. 1998;280:533-8.
31. Kjos SL. Postpartum care of women with diabetes. *Clin Obstet Gynecol.* 2000;43:75-86.

3

Iodine Metabolism in Pregnancy

Maria Thomas, Jubbin J Jacob

INTRODUCTION

Iodine, an essential micronutrient, occurs naturally as its iodide compound and can be found in sea water, marine plants, and soil. Iodide ions in sea water are oxidized and subsequently volatilized in the atmosphere and return to the soil by rain, thus, completing the cycle.[1] In regions where iodine cycling is incomplete, the soil, drinking water, and crops grown are iodine depleted. Iodine-deficient soils are common in mountaineous areas (e.g., Himalayan ranges), areas of frequent flooding, and in coastal and island regions,[1] and iodine deficiency disorders are encountered in animals and human populations in these regions. Biological functions of iodine are mainly due to its role in synthesis of thyroid hormones—triiodothyronine (T_3) and thyroxine (T_4). Their physiological roles can be categorized as:

- Early growth and development of most organs, particularly the brain
- Control of metabolic processes in the body.

Iodized salt, fish (marine), seaweed, shellfish, and eggs are the main sources of dietary iodine.[2] In humans, iodine deficiency affects all ages (*in utero* to the elderly); however, children younger than 3 years, women of reproductive age, pregnant women, and lactating women are particularly susceptible.[3] Severe iodine deficiency within populations results in various disorders ranging from endemic goiter, hypothyroidism, cretinism, decreased fertility rates, increased rates of spontaneous abortions, increased infant mortality, and mental retardation.[4] Mild or asymptomatic maternal hypothyroidism can also cause neurocognitive and psychomotor deficits in the offspring.[5] The World Health Organization (WHO) has reported that 'iodine deficiency is the single, most important, preventable cause of brain damage'.[6] Therefore, population assessment of iodine deficiency and supplementation to improve the iodine status especially among women of childbearing age, pregnant and lactating women, and children, is mandatory.

IODINE PHYSIOLOGY

The dietary iodine is first reduced to iodide, which is then absorbed from the stomach and the duodenum (absorption is >90% in healthy adults).[7] Transporters, such as the sodium iodide symporters located in the apical side of enterocytes and basolateral membrane of thyroid gland, help in active absorption and glandular concentration of iodide.[8] The dietary iodide entering the blood stream rapidly mixes with iodide derived from peripheral catabolism of iodotyrosines to form the extrathyroidal pool of plasma inorganic iodide (PII). PII is in dynamic equilibrium with the thyroid gland and the kidneys. While the renal excretion of iodine is fairly constant (normally >90% of ingested iodine), the uptake by the thyroid gland depends on the dietary intake and the functional state of the thyroid. In a nonpregnant adult, when the iodine intake is adequate (~150 μg/day), the thyroid gland takes up 5–10% of the absorbed iodine. The half-life of plasma iodine is approximately 10 hours in state of adequate iodine intake, whereas in chronic iodine deficiency, the uptake by the thyroid is as high as 80%, and plasma half-life of iodine is greatly shortened.[9] During lactation, the mammary glands also concentrate iodine, which is then secreted in the milk in order to meet iodine demands of newborn.[10] After metabolic equilibrium is achieved, the body maintains an adequate store of iodine in the thyroid ranging between 10 and 20 mg.[11]

In the thyroid sodium iodide symporter concentrates iodide from the serum at a concentration gradient, 20–50 times that of plasma.[12]

Enzymes, such as thyroperoxidase (TPO) and hydrogen peroxide, located at the apical surface of the thyrocyte, oxidize iodide and attach it to the tyrosine residues of thyroglobulin (Tg) to produce monoiodotyrosine (MIT) and diiodotyrosine (DIT), which are then coupled to form T_4 and T_3.[13] Hormone containing Tg is stored in the follicular lumen and when needed, after endocytosis, endosomal and proteosomal lysosomal enzymes, such as cathepsin, causes proteolysis and digestion of Tg to release T_4 and T_3 into the circulation, while DIT and MIT are retained and deiodinated for recycling within the thyroid.[1]

IODINE METABOLISM IN PREGNANCY

Metabolically, pregnancy represents a different steady state as compared to preconception stage. To meet the increased metabolic requirements of pregnancy, the maternal thyroid hormone production needs to be increased by nearly 50%, and hence an increased requirement for iodine that has to be obtained primarily from the diet or as dietary supplements. The increased requirement for thyroid hormone synthesis is attributable to the following causes (Figure 3-1):

- In the early part of the first trimester, there is an increased maternal thyroid hormone production in response to marked increase in serum thyroxine-binding

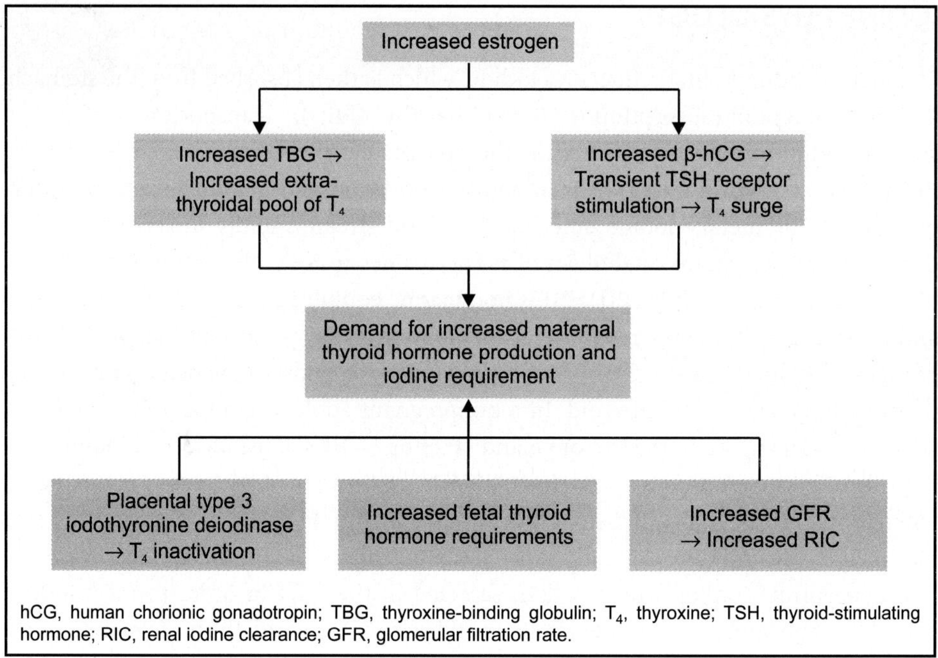

Figure 3-1 Increased thyroid hormone requirement in pregnancy.

globulin (TBG) under the influence of high estrogen concentration. Near the end of the first trimester, there is an increased stimulation of thyroid-stimulating hormone (TSH) receptors by high circulating levels of β-human chorionic gonadotropin (hCG).[11] This is to maintain maternal euthyroidism and to ensure adequate transfer of thyroid hormone to the fetus, as the fetal thyroid does not develop until 13–15 weeks of gestation[14]

- During the second half of gestation, there is an enhanced degradation of T_4 by placental type 3 iodothyronine deiodinase to inactive reverse T_3.[15] Low levels of T_4 trigger TSH secretion by the pituitary, which in turn stimulates thyroid to produce and release more T_4
- Increased renal blood flow and glomerular filtration rate (GFR) early in pregnancy results in 30–50% increase in the renal iodide clearance, and this decreases the circulating PII and, in turn, induces a compensatory increase in the thyroidal clearance of iodide[16] to maintain adequate stores of iodine within the thyroid
- By second half of pregnancy, the fetal thyroid begins hormone synthesis and is totally dependent on the iodide from maternal iodide reserves, which readily cross the placenta.

Because of all the above reasons (Figure 3-1), dietary iodine requirement is much higher in pregnancy as compared to nonpregnant women.[17] A rough estimate of iodine requirement in pregnancy and the daily iodine intake to meet this requirement was made based on the studies that assessed the effect of iodine supplementation with changes in thyroid volume during pregnancy. The WHO, United Nations Children's Fund (UNICEF), and International Council for the Control of Iodine Deficiency Disorders (ICCIDD) recommend a daily iodine intake of 150 μg for nonpregnant, non-lactating adolescents, and adults and 250 μg for pregnant and lactating women.[6]

When the iodine intake is adequate (150 μg/day in a nonpregnant, non-lactating adult), the thyroid stores about 15–20 mg of iodine. When this adult gets pregnant, these stores are sufficient for the gland to adjust its hormonal output to meet the increased demands and to maintain hormone output till pregnancy is complete.

However, when iodine intake is restricted in the preconception stage, the pituitary-thyroid feedback mechanism causes increased iodine trapping in an effort to maintain absolute iodine intake. However, because of the ongoing nutritional deficiency, despite high fractional clearance of PII by the gland, absolute intake falls and stores are depleted further. Pregnancy in a woman with such depleted stores results in a negative iodine balance within the thyroid. In this situation, adequate physiological adaptation cannot be achieved and is replaced by pathological alterations; the severity depending on degree and duration of iodine deprivation.[17]

The consequences of these pathological alterations are relative hypothyroxinemia, secretion of T_3 instead of T_4, increased circulating levels of serum TSH and Tg, and glandular hyperplasia.[18] The fetal thyroid tissue is also extremely sensitive to maternal iodine deprivation and can result in fetal glandular hyperplasia starting in the very early stages of gland development.[11]

ROLE OF IODINE NUTRITION IN PREGNANCY

Dietary iodine intake of approximately 150 μg/day ensures adequate stores, which are sufficient to meet the requirement for increased hormonal output to support the mother and fetus at least in the first trimester. Although the fetal thyroid tissue begins hormone synthesis by beginning of second trimester, the nuclear receptors for thyroid hormones start appearing in the fetal brain as early as 8–9 weeks of gestation, reaching adult levels by 18 weeks.[19] The early appearance of these nuclear receptors facilitates thyroid hormone-dependent neurodevelopment that begins by second half of the first trimester and during this time, cerebral T_3 is generated in the fetal brain by the type II 5'-iodothyronine deiodinase from maternal free T_4.[20] As gestation progresses, the fetus produces increasing amounts of T_4, but the reserves of fetal gland are low, as the gland is still immature and unable to concentrate iodine effectively. At this stage, the amount of hormone produced is insufficient to meet the fetal requirements and the maternal thyroid hormones continue to contribute to the total fetal thyroid hormone concentrations until birth. Fetal neurodevelopment that is dependent on adequate supply of maternal T_4 begins from the second half of the first trimester, and this stage includes neuronal proliferation and migration in the cerebral cortex and the hippocampus. The second stage of neurodevelopment, which is also hormone-dependent, includes axonal growth, dendritic branching, formation of synapses and glial differentiation, and myelin formation.[19]

FETAL-NEONATAL CONSEQUENCES OF MATERNAL IODINE DEFICIENCY AND THYROID IMPAIRMENT

In the initial stages of nutritional deficiency of iodine, the pregnant woman remains euthyroid whereas the fetus develops hypothyroidism. The euthyroid status of the mother is attributed to:

- High circulating levels of β-hCG during pregnancy, which stimulate the TSH receptors and result in a transient free T_4 surge at the end of the first trimester. The thyroid-pituitary feedback, in turn, depresses the concentration of maternal TSH
- Maternal thyroid gland responds to iodine deficiency by increased iodide trapping, preferential synthesis of T_3 over T_4, glandular hyperplasia, and goiter. Due to these reasons, the mother appears euthyroid with TSH and T_3 concentrations fall in the normal range.[21]

In chronic iodine deficiency, the iodine stored is already depleted as a woman enters pregnancy, and hence there is very little iodine available to meet the increased maternal thyroid hormone requirement. This leads to maternal and fetal hypothyroxinemia very early in gestation (Figure 3-2).[21]

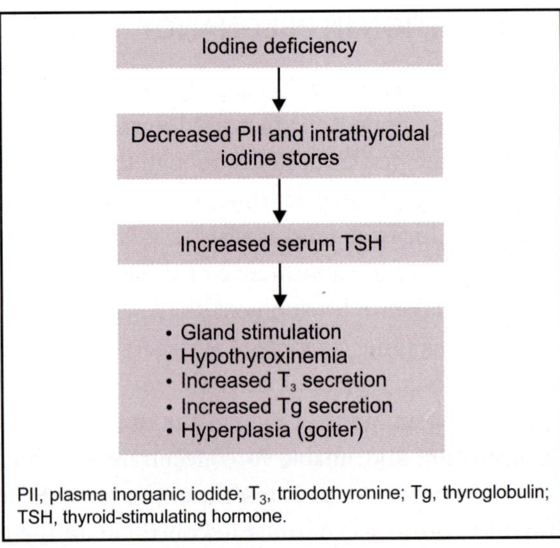

Figure 3-2 Thyroid function in iodine deficient states.

The fetus being solely dependent on maternal thyroid hormone for its neurodevelopment during gestation and early postnatal life, the hypothyroxinemia during these critical periods causes irreversible brain damage with neuro-psycho-intellectual impairment, mental retardation, and neurological abnormalities;[22] the severity depending upon the timing and degree of the hypothyroxinemia.

The prevalence of attention deficit and hyperactivity disorders is higher in the offsprings of women living in mild-to-moderate iodine-deficient areas than those in iodine-replete regions.[5] Intelligence quotient (IQ) levels of children living in severely iodine-deficient areas are an average of 12.45 points lower than those living in iodine-replete areas and are improved with iodine supplementation.[23] In women of childbearing age, severe iodine deficiency and hypothyroidism result in reduced fertility and increased rates of spontaneous abortions.[11]

IODINE SUPPLEMENTATION DURING PREGNANCY

Maternal iodine deficiency results in neurodevelopmental damage in the fetus leading to mental retardation in the progeny, which could have been prevented by adequate iodine supplementation.

Iodine supplementation programs should target the diet of the whole population, especially, women in the childbearing age in whom iodine supplementation should ideally start long before pregnancy. It is done to facilitate reaching a long-term steady state with plentiful iodine stores in the thyroid gland so that they have no difficulty adapting to the increased demand of the thyroid hormones during pregnancy[24] or as soon as possible during gestation and continue supplementation after parturition for women who are breastfeeding.

Salt Fortification with Iodine

In 1993, WHO and UNICEF recommended universal salt iodization as the most cost-effective way of delivering iodine and of improving cognition in iodine-deficient populations.[25] Universal salt iodization ensures that all salt for human and animal consumption be adequately iodized and has been effective in most countries. Iodine concentration in salt at the point of production should be within the range of 20–40 mg of iodine per kg of salt (i.e., 20–40 ppm of iodine) in order to provide 150 μg of iodine per person per day (corresponds to a median urinary iodine levels varying between 100 and 200 μg/L).[6] Iodine can be added to salt in the form of potassium iodide or potassium iodate, but latter is preferred to iodide, because it is much more stable in the presence of impurities, humidity, and porous packing and is the recommended form in tropical countries and those with low grade salt.[6]

Despite fortification, several factors can result in up to 80% loss of iodine; hence, it is important to have regular surveys of the median iodine urinary levels carried out in a sample of the at-risk population to ensure adequate iodization.[6]

TABLE 3-1

Recommended Dosages of Daily and Annual Iodine Supplementation (WHO 2007)		
Population subgroup	*Daily dose of Iodine supplement (µg/dL)*	*Single annual dose of iodized oil supplement (mg/year)*
Pregnant women	250	400
Lactating women	250	400
Women in reproductive age (15–49 years)	150	400

Source: WHO, UNICEF, ICCIDD. Assessment of the iodine deficiency disorders and monitoring their elimination. Geneva (Switzerland): World Health Organization. Available from: http://whqlibdoc.who.int/publication/2007/9789241595827_eng.pdf.2007.

Iodine Supplementation

In certain regions where availability of iodized salt is not practical, other options for correction of iodine deficiency are available. These include administration of iodized oil supplements either orally or as intramuscular injections. Intramuscular injections have a longer duration of action, but oral route is preferred because of ease of administration. Iodized oil is prepared by esterification of unsaturated fatty acids in seed or vegetable oils and addition of iodine to the double bonds. Usual doses are 200–400 mg in iodine per year,[6] and the target population is women of childbearing age, pregnant women,[26] and children (Table 3-1).

Iodine solutions, such as Lugol's iodine, containing 6 mg iodine per drop at regular intervals (once a month is sufficient) and potassium iodide or potassium iodate tablets or drops can also be used as supplements. Single oral doses of potassium iodide monthly (30 mg) or biweekly (8 mg) can provide adequate iodine for school-age children.[27] Prenatal multivitamin preparations containing iodine (~150 µg/day) are also available. In multivitamin supplements containing iodine, the actual iodine content is not determined by the original amount added but also by the stability of the compound, the time elapsed since manufacture, and the conditions under which the product is stored.

Kelp and seaweed-based products, because of unacceptable variability in their iodine content, should be avoided, and it has been reported that daily dose was greater than 1100 µg/day, much greater than the recommended safe upper limit for pregnancy.[28]

ASSESSMENT OF IODINE STATUS DURING PREGNANCY

Indicators are used to assess baseline iodine status and to monitor and evaluate the response of the population to iodine supplementation. Four methods available for assessment of thyroid nutrition in population are:

- Urinary iodine concentration
- TSH levels

- Tg
- Assessment of thyroid size/volume by palpation/ultrasonography.

These indicators are complementary, i.e., urinary iodine concentration is a sensitive indicator of recent iodine intake (days) and Tg shows an intermediate response (weeks to months), whereas changes in the thyroid size rate reflect long-term iodine nutrition (months to years).[1]

Urinary Iodine Concentration

As 90% of ingested iodine is excreted in the urine, urinary iodine concentration is a widely used method for assessment of iodine status, and it reflects recent changes in iodine intake or administration.[1,6] Urinary iodine values from population are not normally distributed due to variability in its excretion. Hence, the median urinary iodine concentration is used in population surveys to assess the iodine nutrition among pregnant and lactating women and young children of less than 2 years of age.[6] Although urinary iodine concentration is used as an indicator of iodine intake, median urinary iodine concentration does not provide direct information about thyroid function. However, a low median urinary iodine concentration indicates that a population is at risk of developing thyroid disorders.[1]

Daily iodine intake in adults can be extrapolated from the urinary iodine concentration assuming 24 hours urine volume of 1.5 L, iodine bioavailability of 92%, and urinary excretion of iodine approaching 90%, using the formula:[1]

$$\text{Urinary iodine } (\mu g/L) \times 0.0235 \times \text{Body weight (kg)} = \text{Daily iodine intake}$$

Using this formula, a median urinary iodine of 100 μg/L corresponds roughly to an average daily intake of 150 μg.[28] Using this estimation, a urinary iodine of 140 μg/L would correspond to a daily intake of 200 μg/L iodine. However, during pregnancy, due to increase in GFR and renal clearance of iodine, this extrapolation is less valid and the daily iodine intake extrapolated from the urinary iodine concentration in pregnancy would be lower than that in nonpregnancy. A recent WHO expert group recommended the median urinary iodine that indicates adequate iodine intake during pregnancy to be 150–249 μg/L (Table 3-2).[6] However, these are population indicators and should not be used for individual diagnosis and treatment.

The urinary iodine concentration (μg/L) is not interchangeable with 24 hours urinary iodine excretion (μg per 24 hours). The two values are interchangeable only, if the volume of urine passed in 24 hours is 1 liter. However, since an adult passes approximately 1.5 L per 24 hours of urine, the median urinary iodine excretion given as μg per 24 hours will be 50% higher than the median iodine excretion given as μg/L.

With universal salt iodization, there have been reports of excessive iodization, which may lead to iodine induced hyperthyroidism and autoimmune diseases and, therefore, even in iodine deficient populations, excessive supplementation with iodine (i.e., urinary iodine concentration >200 μg/L) is not recommended.[28]

TABLE 3-2

Epidemiological Criteria for Assessing Iodine Nutrition Based on the Median or Range in Urinary Iodine Concentrations of Pregnant Women[a]		
Population subgroup	*Median urinary iodine concentration (μg/L)*	*Iodine intake*
Pregnant women	<150	Insufficient
	≥150–249	Adequate
	250–499	Above requirements
	500	Excessive[b]

[a]For lactating women and children <2 years of age, a median urinary iodine concentration of 100 μg/L can be used to define adequate iodine intake. Although lactating women have the same requirement as pregnant women, the median urinary iodine is lower because iodine is excreted in breast milk.
[b]The term "excessive" means in excess of the amount required to prevent and control iodine deficiency.
Source: WHO, UNICEF, ICCIDD, Assessment of the iodine deficiency disorders and monitoring their elimination. Geneva (Switzerland): World Health Organization. Available from: http://whqlibdoc.who.int/publication/2007/9789241595827_eng.pdf.2007.

Thyroglobulin

Tg is a precursor protein in the production of thyroid hormones and is thyroid specific. Stimulation of thyroid by TSH releases small amounts of Tg from the thyrocytes, which are cleared by the liver.[29] Elevated Tg levels indicate increased thyroid mass, increased TSH stimulation, or thyroid injury.[30] In areas of chronic iodine deficiency, elevated serum Tg reflects thyrotropin hyperstimulation and thyroid hyperplasia; however, their concentrations often remain in normal range and increases over several months. Hence, it reflects iodine nutrition over a period of months or years in contrast to urinary iodine concentration, which assesses more immediate iodine intake.[6] After 42–52 weeks of iodine repletion, Tg shows a positive correlation with thyroid volume and thyrotropin[31] and, hence, seems a valid iodine deficiency disorder indicator as it detects changes in thyroid function in response to changes in iodine supply, which is not shown with urinary iodine.[32] In population studies, the serum Tg concentration is a good marker of iodine, but a high serum concentration of Tg is not a specific sign of iodine deficiency as even in iodine replete state, any stimulation of thyroid will lead to an increase in the serum concentration of Tg. During a normal pregnancy, there is a considerable increase in requirements for thyroid hormone and, therefore, also in thyroid secretory activity.[33] Findings of a study from Denmark suggested that the increase in serum Tg concentration during pregnancy is primarily caused by greater thyroid secretory activity and that, it is not a sign of iodine deficiency.[34]

Thyroid-stimulating Hormone Assessment

In states of iodine deficiency, serum TSH and Tg takes several weeks to rise and often remain in the euthyroid range. Hence, they are not good indicators of iodine deficiency.[22] A higher concentration of TSH and Tg in cord blood as compared to maternal blood is not a sign of iodine deficiency in the mother or neonate. This is a normal phenomenon, not related to iodine deficiency and the difference remains even after iodine supplementation.[35]

CONCLUSION

During pregnancy, there is an increased thyroid hormone requirement, which is met by a 50% increase in hormone production by the thyroid gland. Increased production, in turn, depends upon the availability of iodine either in the diet or as supplements.

When there is a deficiency of iodine, adequate adaptation to the new physiological state is not possible, and it results in pathological alterations like glandular hyperplasia. Maternal and fetal hypothyroxinemia results depending upon the timing, duration, and degree of iodine deprivation. Iodine deficiency during pregnancy also results in impaired neuropsychological development leading to neurologic and psychological deficits in the progeny. IQ levels of children living in severely iodine-deficient areas are an average of 12.45 points lower than those living in iodine-replete areas and are improved with iodine supplementation. It is, therefore, important to assess presence and degree of iodine deficiency in a population. Iodine supplementation should be given to all women of childbearing age, pregnant and lactating mothers, and children. Iodine supplementation has proved highly beneficial in preventing mental disorders.

The Indian Thyroid Society (ITS) guidelines for management of thyroid dysfunction during pregnancy recommend early diagnosis of maternal hypothyroidism, preferably at the first prenatal visit or at the time of diagnosis of pregnancy, based on trimester-specific TSH and low T_4 values, and close monitoring at regular intervals till adequate and appropriate adjustment is achieved.[36]

However, pregnant women from iodine-replete areas have adequate stores of iodine in the thyroid gland and do not require routine supplementation. If supplementation is needed, iodized salt as the preferred mode of delivery for correction of iodine deficiency disorders has been recommended by ITS guidelines.[37]

Regular surveys of salt iodine content and urinary iodine levels should be carried out to determine if the program is having the desired effect. WHO has issued criteria for assessing iodine nutrition based on the median or range in urinary iodine concentrations of pregnant women in a population.

REFERENCES

1. Zimmermann MB. Iodine deficiency. *Endocr Rev*. 2009;30:376-408.
2. Human Vitamin and Mineral Requirements. Report of a joint FAO/WHO expert consultation Bangkok, Thailand. 2001. p. 181-94.

3. WHO Secretariat, Andersson M, de Benoist B, Delange F, Zupan J. Prevention and control of iodine deficiency in pregnant and lactating women and in children less than 2-years-old: conclusions and recommendations of the Technical Consultation. *Public Health Nutr.* 2007;10:1606-11.
4. Perez-Lopez FR. Iodine and thyroid hormones during pregnancy and postpartum. *Gynecol Endocrino.* 2007;23:414-28.
5. Vermiglio F, Lo Presti VP, Moleti M, Sidoti M, Tortorella G, Scaffidi G, et al. Attention deficit and hyperactivity disorders in the offspring of mothers exposed to mild-moderate iodine deficiency: a possible novel iodine deficiency disorder in developed countries. *J Clin Endocrinol Metab.* 2004;89:6054-60.
6. WHO, UNICEF, ICCIDD. Assessment of the iodine deficiency disorders and monitoring their elimination. Geneva (Switzerland): World Health Organization. Available from: http://whqlibdoc.who.int/publication/2007/9789241595827_eng.pdf.2007.
7. Alexander WD, Harden RM, Harrison MT, Shimmins J. Some aspects of the absorption and concentration of iodide by the alimentary tract in man. *Proc Nutr Soc.* 1967;26:62-6.
8. Nicola JP, Basquin C, Portulano C, Reyna-Neyra A, Paroder M, Carrasco N. The Na_/I-symporter mediates active iodide uptake in the intestine. *Am J Physiol Cell Physiol.* 2009;296:C654-62.
9. DeGroot LJ Kinetic analysis of iodine metabolism. *J Clin Endocrinol Metab.*1966;26:149-73.
10. Weaver JC, Kamm ML, Dobson RL. 1960 Excretion of radioiodine in human milk. *J Am Med Asso.* 1960;173:872-5.
11. Glinoer D. The importance of iodine nutrition during pregnancy. *Public Health Nutr.* 2007;10:1542-6.
12. Eskandari S, Loo DD, Dai G, Levy O, Wright EM, Carrasco N. Thyroid Na^+/I- symporter. Mechanism, stoichiometry, and specificity. *J Biol Chem.* 1997;272:27230-8.
13. Dunn JT. Thyroglobulin, hormone synthesis and thyroid disease. *Eur J Endocrinol.* 1995; 132:603-4.
14. Glioner D. The Regulation of Thyroid Function in Pregnancy: Pathways of Endocrine Adaptation from Physiology to Pathology. *Endocr Rev.* 1997;18:404-33.
15. Roti E, Fang SL, Emerson CH, Braverman LE. Placental inner ring iodothyronine deiodination: a mechanism for decreased passage of T_4 and T_3 from mother to fetus. *Trans Assoc Am Physicians.* 1981;94:183-9.
16. Dafnis E, Sabatini S. The effect of pregnancy on renal function: physiology and pathophysiology. *Am J Med Sci.* 1992;303:184-205.
17. Glinoer D. Pregnancy and iodine. *Thyroid.* 2001;11:471-81.
18. Glinoer D. Maternal and fetal impact of chronic iodine deficiency. *Clin Obstet Gynecol.* 1997;40:102-16.
19. Williams GR. Neurodevelopmental and neurophysiological actions of thyroid hormones. *J Neuroendocrinol.* 2008;20:784-94.
20. Skeaff SA. Iodine Deficiency in Pregnancy: The Effect on Neurodevelopment in the Child. *Nutrients.* 2011;3:265-73.
21. de Escobar GM, Obregón MJ, del Rey FE. Maternal thyroid hormones early in pregnancy and fetal brain development. *Best Pract Res Clin Endocrinol Metab.* 2004;18:225-48.
22. Leung AM, Pearce EN, Braverman LE. Iodine Nutrition in Pregnancy and Lactation. *Endocrinol Metab Clin North Am.* 2011;40:765-77.

23. Qian M, Wang D, Watkins WE, Gebski V, Yan YQ, Li M, et al. The effects of iodine on intelligence in children: a metaanalysis of studies conducted in China. *Asia Pac J Clin Nutr.* 2005;14:32-42.
24. Liberman CS, Pino SC, Fang SL, Braverman LE, Emerson CH. Circulating iodide concentrations during and after pregnancy. *J Clin Endocrinol Metab.* 1998;83:3545-9.
25. Engle PL, Black MM, Behrman JR, Cabral de Mello M, Gertler PJ, Kapiriri L, et al. International Child Development Steering Group. Strategies to avoid the loss of developmental potential in more than 200 million children in the developing world. *Lancet.* 2007;369:229-42.
26. Delange F. Administration of iodized oil during pregnancy: a summary of the published evidence. *Bull World Health Organ.*1996;74:101-8.
27. Todd CH, Dunn JT. Intermittent oral administration of potassium iodide solution for the correction of iodine deficiency. *Am J Clin Nutr.* 1998;67:1279-83.
28. Institute of Medicine, Academy of Sciences. Dietary reference intakes for vitamin A, Vitamin K, arsenic, boron, chromium, copper, iodine, iron, manganese, molybdenum, nickel, silicon, vanadium, and zinc. Washington, DC:National Academy Press; 2001. p. 258-89.
29. Tórrens JI, Burch HB. Serum thyroglobulin measurement. *Endocrinol Metab Clin North Am.* 2001;30:429-67.
30. Spencer CA. Thyroglobulin measurement: techniques, clinical benefits, and pitfalls. *Endocrinol Metab Clin North Am.* 1995;24:841-63.
31. Bascheri L, Pinchera A. Reciprocal changes of serum thyroglobulin and TSH in residents of a moderate endemic goitre area. *Clin Endocrinol.* 1985;23:115-22.
32. Zimmermann M, Adou P, Torresani T, Zeder C, Hurrell R. Low dose oral iodized oil for control of iodine deficiency in children. *Br J Nutr.* 2000;84:139-41.
33. Feldt-Rasmussen, U. Serum thyroglobulin and thyroglobulin autoantibodies in thyroid diseases. Pathogenic and diagnostic aspects. *Allergy.* 1983;38:369-87.
34. Laurberg P, Andersen S, Bjarnadóttir RI, Carlé A, Hreidarsson A, Knudsen N, et al. Evaluating iodine deficiency in pregnant women and young infants—complex physiology with a risk of misinterpretation. *Public Health Nutr.* 2007;10:1547-52.
35. Pedersen KM, Laurberg P, Iversen E, Knudsen PR, Gregersen HE, Rasmussen OS, et al. Amelioration of some pregnancy associated variations in thyroid function by iodine supplementation. *J Clin Endocrinol Metab.* 1993;77:1078-83.
36. Guidelines for Management of Thyroid Dysfunction During Pregnancy. An Initiative from Indian Thyroid Society. Endorsed by- Endocrine Society of India. 2012. p. 2-6.
37. Guidelines for Management of Thyroid Dysfunction During Pregnancy. An Initiative from Indian Thyroid Society. Endorsed by- Endocrine Society of India. 2012. p. 23-4.

4

Hypothyroidism and Pregnancy

Rajesh Rajput

INTRODUCTION

Hypothyroidism occurs commonly in the reproductive age group and is a well-recognized complication of pregnancy and puerperium. Various screening studies have shown that overt hypothyroidism is estimated to occur in 0.3–0.5% of pregnancies while subclinical hypothyroidism appears to occur in 2–3% of all pregnancies.[1] The etiology of hypothyroidism during pregnancy is not different from that in nonpregnant women. In iodine replete areas, Hashimoto's thyroiditis is the leading cause, while in iodine deficient areas, iodine deficiency itself is the most common cause of hypothyroidism. The various other less common causes include overtreatment of hyperthyroidism, concomitant use of various medications that alter the absorption of levothyroxine (LT_4), and various pituitary and hypothalamic disorders.[2,3]

NORMAL PHYSIOLOGY

Several alterations in thyroid physiology occur during various stages of pregnancy, which are completely reversible in the postpartum period. The most common alterations in thyroid physiology are increase in thyroid binding globulin (TBG), increase in glomerular filtration rate (GFR) resulting in increased iodide clearance, transplacental transfer of thyroxine (T_4) and iodine for normal fetal brain development, and increased placental degradation of thyroid hormones (Figure 4-1). As a result of these physiological adaptations, maternal thyroid hormone production increases and results in elevation of total triiodothyronine (T_3) and T_4 levels in normal pregnant women. If this compensation is inadequate or absent, it results in clinical or subclinical hypothyroidism during pregnancy.[2,3]

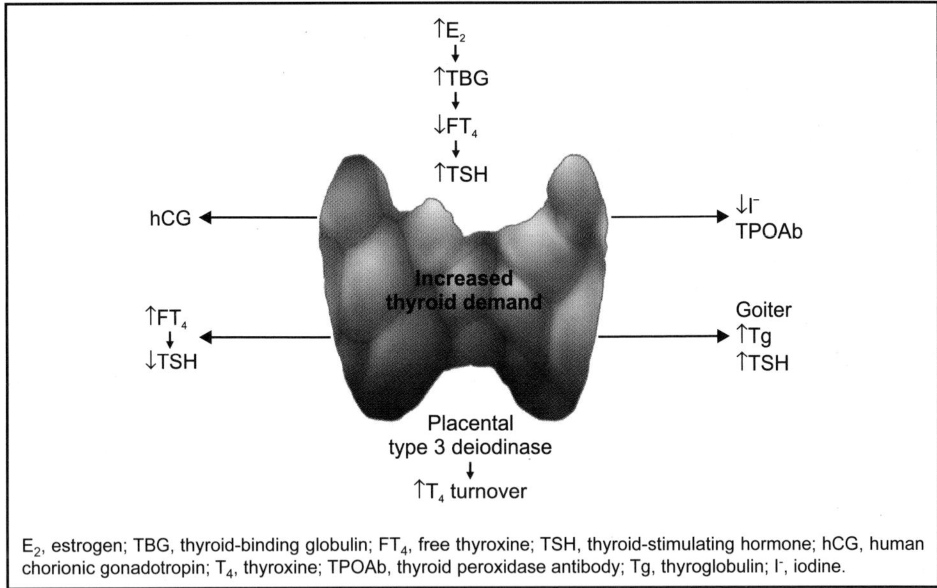

Figure 4-1 Normal physiological alterations in thyroid functions during pregnancy.

EFFECT OF HYPOTHYROIDISM ON PREGNANCY OUTCOMES

Untreated hypothyroidism in the mother may cause microcytic anemia, preeclampsia, placental abruption, postpartum hemorrhage, and miscarriage.[4] Subclinical hypothyroidism has also been associated with spontaneous abortion and preterm labor.[4,5]

FETAL AND NEONATAL CONSEQUENCES OF MATERNAL HYPOTHYROIDISM

Before fetal thyroid gland starts functioning, the fetus is solely dependent on maternal iodine and T_4 transfer across the placenta for normal neuropsychological development. If maternal hypothyroidism is not recognized early in pregnancy, it may result in serious consequences ranging from decrease in intelligent quotient (IQ) to frank mental retardation. Development of fetal brain with neuronal multiplication, migration, and architectural organization occurs during first and second trimesters and is almost exclusively dependent on maternal T_4 levels. The later phases of brain development like glial cell multiplication, migration, and myelinization occur largely during third trimester and during first 3 years of life. It is dependent on fetal and neonatal thyroid hormone synthesis. Therefore, severe maternal hypothyroidism developing early during pregnancy results in irreversible brain damage. Maternal hypothyroidism developing during later part of gestation results in less severe and also partially reversible brain damage.[6,7]

AUTOIMMUNE THYROID DISORDERS AND PREGNANCY

Pregnancy is characterized by elevation of progesterone and estradiol levels with overall increase in their ratio. The elevated progesterone decreases reactivity of both humoral and cellular arms of the immune system while estradiol exerts opposite effect. Apart from these hormonal alterations, several, not well elucidated, mechanisms result in partial immune tolerance during pregnancy which reverts back in the postpartum period. This results in an increased chance of thyroiditis during postpartum period.[8]

The presence of thyroid autoimmunity as characterized by elevated thyroid peroxidase antibody (TPOAb) levels in an otherwise euthyroid pregnant woman is found to be associated with adverse pregnancy consequences, including increased fetal loss in various studies. The reason behind this association is not clearly established, but various likely reasons include the following:

- Thyroid autoimmunity representing an underlying, more generalized immune imbalance that results in greater rejection of the fetus rather than elevated TPOAb levels causing it directly
- Lesser ability of diseased thyroid gland to adapt to physiological changes associated with pregnancy, resulting in reduced functional thyroid reserve despite apparently normal thyroid functions
- Women of advanced age becoming pregnant with underlying thyroid autoimmunity.[9]

Pregnant women who are otherwise positive for thyroid autoimmunity and had normal thyroid function tests initially, show gradual decline in parameters of thyroid functions despite apparent decrease in titers of TPOAb as gestation advances. As a result of this, as much as 50% of pregnant women have low normal or subnormal T_4 levels, indicating the need for timely detection and intervention in such women. Whether all these women should be treated with LT_4 is not clear at present, but if a pregnant woman is having thyroid-stimulating hormone (TSH) levels of more than 2.0 mIU/L with TPOAb more than 12500 U/mL before 20 weeks of gestation, the chances of progression to subclinical/overt hypothyroidism are very high before the end of pregnancy. Such cases should be closely followed up during their gestation and in the postpartum period.[10] Several recent clinical trials have shown beneficial effects of LT_4 on pregnancy outcomes in such women irrespective of their baseline thyroid status.[11]

DIAGNOSIS

For diagnosing hypothyroidism during pregnancy, one should use trimester-specific cutoff for thyroid function tests and should order free T_3 and free T_4 rather than total T_3 and T_4 in view of increased TBG levels during pregnancy. If facility for measurement of free T_3 and free T_4 is not available, one should then adjust the increased thyroid hormone production during pregnancy by multiplying the normal nonpregnant range for total T_4 by a factor of 1.5 during pregnancy. Trimester specific cutoff is well established for TSH but not for serum free T_4 levels. The normal range for TSH during pregnancy is 0.1–2.5 mIU/L during first trimester and 0.2–3.0 mIU/L during second and third trimesters. In primary hypothyroidism, TSH levels are elevated and free T_4 should be low, while in secondary or tertiary hypothyroidism, TSH levels are low or normal in presence of low free T_4. Subclinical hypothyroidism is diagnosed in the presence of normal free T_4 and elevated TSH levels.[12]

TREATMENT

LT_4 is the drug of choice for treatment of subclinical and overt hypothyroidism during pregnancy. The dose of LT_4 depends on the severity of thyroid derangement and the timing of diagnosis. For newly diagnosed patient, it should be started in a dose of 2 µg/kg body weight, which is slightly higher than what is used in nonpregnant women. The drug has to be taken empty stomach, and at least 4 hours before any iron or calcium supplementation is taken by pregnant women. If these precautions are not taken, the absorption of LT_4 decreases by as much as 20–30% resulting in poor control of disease as well as injudicious increase in the dosage. The thyroid function should be rechecked after every 4 weeks to adjust the dosage, if needed. The objective is to keep TSH below 2.5 mIU/L during the first trimester and below 3.0 mIU/L during the second and third trimesters. For previously diagnosed hypothyroid women becoming pregnant, the need for LT_4 increases by as much as 30–50% during gestation as a result of number of physiological alterations already discussed. For such women, the dose of LT_4 should be increased depending on their baseline thyroid function test with the aim of maintaining TSH below 2.5 mIU/L during the first trimester and below 3.0 mIU/L during the second and third trimesters (Table 4-1).

TABLE 4-1

Levothyroxine Dosage for Various Baseline TSH Levels	
Baseline TSH levels (mIU/L)	*LT_4 Dosage (µg/day)*
TSH <10	Increase by 50
TSH 10–20	Increase by 75
TSH >20	Increase by 100

TSH, thyroid-stimulating hormone; LT_4, levothyroxine.

Thyroid function test should be reassessed at least 4 weeks after any modification in the dosage. Once thyroid function is in the normal range for pregnancy, repeat thyroid function tests should be done every 6 weeks. The recommended mean intake of iodine during pregnancy and lactation is approximately 250 μg/day.[13-15]

American Thyroid Association Recommendations

In the year 2011, American Thyroid Association (ATA) issued its recommendations regarding the diagnosis and management of thyroid disorders during pregnancy, highlighting the role of thyroid function tests, thyrotoxicosis, hypothyroidism, iodine, thyroid antibodies, miscarriage/preterm delivery, thyroid nodules and cancer, postpartum thyroiditis, various recommendations for screening for thyroid diseases in pregnancy, and areas for future research.[16] The specific recommendations relating to hypothyroidism and pregnancy are summarized in table 4-2.

Indian Thyroid Society Recommendations

Recently, Indian Thyroid Society (ITS)[17] has also given its recommendations for diagnosis and management of hypothyroidism in pregnancy, and they are not very

TABLE 4-2

ATA Recommendations for Hypothyroidism During Pregnancy
• Oral LT_4 is indicated for women with overt hypothyroidism, which is associated with greater risks for fetal loss and premature birth and for those with subclinical hypothyroidism who are positive for TPOAb
• To treat maternal hypothyroidism, use of T_3, desiccated thyroid, or other thyroid preparations is strongly recommended against
• Women who are already receiving thyroid replacement therapy should increase their dose by 25–30% when they become pregnant
• Women with subclinical hypothyroidism initially untreated in pregnancy should be monitored for disease advancement to overt hypothyroidism. Serum TSH and free T_4 levels should be measured every 4 weeks, approximately, until 16–20 weeks of gestation, and at least once between 26 and 32 weeks of gestation
• In the first trimester, normal range for TSH level is 0.1–2.5 mIU/L; this level increases to 0.2–3.0 mIU/L in the second trimester and 0.3–3.0 mIU/L in the third trimester
• Serum levels of free T_4 during pregnancy should be measured with online solid-phase extraction liquid chromatography or tandem mass spectrometry on serum dialysate or ultrafiltrate
• Treatment is not needed for women with low isolated free T_4 levels.

ATA, American Thyroid Association; LT_4, levothyroxine; TPOAb, thyroid peroxidase antibody; TSH, thyroid-stimulating hormone; T_4, thyroxine; T_3, triiodothyronine.

Source: Stagnaro-green A, Abalovich M, Alexander E, Azizi F, Mestman J, Negro R, et al. Guidelines of American Thyroid Association for Diagnosis and Management of Thyroid disease during pregnancy and postpartum. *Thyroid.* 2011;21:1081-125.

different from ATA recommendations. ITS recommends that diagnosis should be based on trimester-specific TSH and low total T_4. Patients diagnosed with overt hypothyroidism during pregnancy should start the therapy with full replacement dose of LT_4 (1.6–2.0 μg/kg/day) to normalize thyroid function tests as rapidly as possible. Monitoring of treatment should be done by measuring free T_4 and TSH levels every 6 weeks. Subclinical hypothyroidism has been shown to be associated with an adverse outcome for both the mother and offspring and, hence, should be treated with LT_4. The appropriate adjustments in LT_4 dosage should be done to maintain the target TSH levels at less than 2.5 mIU/L in first trimester and 3 mIU/L in the second and third trimesters. Women with preexisting hypothyroidism in whom thyroid assessment cannot be done immediately should have their LT_4 dose increased by 30%, as soon as pregnancy is diagnosed. Post-delivery, the patient should be reverted back to the prepregnant dosage and TSH levels should be rechecked after 6 weeks. Even the women with thyroid autoimmunity who are euthyroid in the early stages of pregnancy are at an increased risk of developing hypothyroidism and should be monitored for TSH every trimester.

SCREENING OF ALL PREGNANT WOMEN FOR HYPOTHYROIDISM

Despite the fact that several studies have suggested brain developmental abnormalities ranging from mild decrease in IQ to mental retardation in children born to women who had subclinical to overt hypothyroidism during pregnancy, there is no general consensus related to the screening of all women for hypothyroidism during pregnancy. However, few groups/associations recommend checking a woman's TSH value either before becoming pregnant, or as soon as pregnancy is confirmed. This holds true for women who are at higher risk for thyroid disease like those with previous treatment for hyperthyroidism, a positive family history of thyroid disease, and those with goiter. Evidently, women having hypothyroidism should undergo a TSH test once pregnancy is confirmed, as the requirements of thyroid hormone surging during pregnancy often leads to an essential increase in the LT_4 dose. If TSH is normal, further monitoring is not typically required.[16,18]

Controversy still surrounds whether or not to screen for postpartum thyroiditis in all women.[16] The American Congress of Obstetricians and Gynecologists (ACOG) does not recommend postpartum thyroid screening. The ATA states that this decision of screening in women of childbearing age should be made mutually between the physician and the patient. The American Association of Clinical Endocrinologists (AACE) recommends that in the pregnant women who are known to have high titers of TPOAb, postpartum screening should be done. In the middle of these controversies, it is recommended to do selective screening based on risk profile of postpartum women,

TABLE 4-3

Women at High Risk for Postpartum Thyroiditis
• Women with type 1 diabetes mellitus or other autoimmune disorders
• Women with a strong family history of autoimmune thyroid disease
• TPOAb-positive
• Prior episode of postpartum thyroiditis
• Postpartum depression
• Women with prior miscarriage.

TPOAb, thyroid peroxidase antibody.

as mentioned in table 4-3. Screening should include TPOAb titers and TSH levels. In euthyroid women and those who are TPOAb-negative, there is no requirement of further follow-up. Women who are TPOAb-positive should undergo a serum TSH examination at 6 and 9 months postpartum.

POSTPARTUM THYROIDITIS

Postpartum thyroiditis occurs in women within first year after the delivery of the baby. It occurs in approximately 5–10% of women, but the incidence can be greater in certain high-risk women as mentioned in table 4-3.[16,19]

Following the partial immunosuppression of pregnancy, there occurs an immunological rebound, which aggravates an underlying autoimmune thyroiditis, thus, leading to postpartum thyroiditis. It may present as transient hyperthyroidism, transient hypothyroidism, or transient hyperthyroidism followed by transient hypothyroidism. The postpartum thyroiditis comprises of thyrotoxicosis followed by hypothyroidism, but it is not evident that all women go through both the phases; while 1/3rd of patients manifest both phases, other patients will manifest only a thyrotoxic or hypothyroid phase.[20]

The thyrotoxic phase usually occurs 1–4 months postpartum, lasts for 1–3 months, and is associated with symptoms, including anxiety, palpitations, insomnia, fatigue, weight loss, and irritability. In majority of women, all the above cited symptoms are often attributed to the postpartum phase and the anxiety of having a new baby. Thus, the thyrotoxic phase of postpartum thyroiditis is often missed. Commonly, women present in the hypothyroid phase, which characteristically occurs 4–8 months postpartum and may last for up to 9–12 months. Typical symptoms include fatigue, weight gain, constipation, dry skin, depression, and poor exercise tolerance. The thyroid function returns to normal within 12–18 months of the onset of symptoms in most of the women.[21]

The choice of treatment primarily depends on the phase of thyroiditis and degree of symptoms exhibited by the patient. β-blockers are administered to decrease palpitations

TABLE 4-4

Recommendations of ITS for Evaluation and Management of Postpartum Thyroiditis
• Routine screening of all women for postpartum thyroiditis is not justified. Women who have type 1 diabetes mellitus or are TPO-positive during the first trimester, should have their TSH monitored at 3 and 6 months postpartum
• Majority of women in the hyperthyroid phase do not require intervention
• Symptomatic cases should be managed with a short course of β-blockers
• Symptomatic women with a TSH >10 mIU/L or between 4 and 10 mIU/L, as well as, asymptomatic women with a TSH between 4 and 10 mIU/L and planning pregnancy in the near future, should be treated with LT_4
• The duration of therapy with LT_4 should be approximately, 1 year postpartum or until the woman completes her family. No clear association between presence of postpartum thyroiditis or thyroid antibodies and postpartum depression has been established
• Women with postpartum depression should be screened for hypothyroidism and treated appropriately.

ITS, Indian Thyroid Society; TPO, thyroid peroxidase antibody; TSH, thyroid-stimulating hormone; LT_4, levothyroxine.

Source: Guidelines for Management of Thyroid Dysfunction During Pregnancy. An Initiative from Indian Thyroid Society. Endorsed by- Endocrine Society of India. 2012; *with permission*.

and others symptoms accompanying hyperthyroidism in women who present with thyrotoxicosis. The medication is tapered off as the symptoms improve, since the thyrotoxic phase is transient. Among β-blockers, propranolol is recommended by the Food and Drug Administration (FDA) as a safe drug to be used during lactation. Antithyroid medications are not indicated for the thyrotoxic phase since the thyroid gland *per se* is not overactive. LT_4 is the choice of treatment for the hypothyroid phase for thyroid hormone replacement. In case of mild hypothyroidism and if the patient has few, if any, symptoms, no therapy may be necessary. If thyroid hormone therapy has begun, treatment should be continued for approximately 6–12 months and then tapered to see if the patient requires thyroid hormone permanently, since approximately 80% of patients regain normal thyroid function and do not require a need for chronic therapy. However, approximately 20% of patients who go into a hypothyroid phase will remain hypothyroid and will require continuation of LT_4 therapy. In women where LT_4 is stopped, serum TSH should be monitored annually for early detection of future hypothyroidism.[19,21] Recommendations given by Indian Thyroid Society[17] for postpartum thyroiditis are summarized in table 4-4.

CONCLUSION

Hypothyroidism is one of the well-known complications of pregnancy and puerperal period. If untreated, it may complicate the normal course of pregnancy by various maternal and fetal conditions like preeclampsia, placental abruption, miscarriage, etc. in the mother; fetal growth and development may also be affected. Thus, adequate screening and early initiation of LT_4 according to the severity of the condition is recommended.

REFERENCES

1. Abalovich M, Amino N, Barbour LA, Cobin RH, De Groot LJ, Glinoer D, et al. Management of thyroid dysfunction during pregnancy and postpartum: an Endocrine Society Clinical Practice Guideline. *J Clin Endocrinol Metab*. 2007;92:S1-47.
2. Becks GP, Burrow GN. Thyroid disease and pregnancy. *Med Clin North Am*. 1991;75: 121-50.
3. LeBeau SO, Mandel SJ. Thyroid disorders during pregnancy. *Endocrinol Metab Clin North Am*. 2006;35:117-36.
4. Poppe K, Velkeniers B, Glinoer D. Thyroid disease and female reproduction. *Clin Endocrinol (Oxf)*. 2007;66:309-21.
5. Cooper DS. Clinical practice. Subclinical hypothyroidism. *N Engl J Med*. 2001;345:260-5.
6. Leung AS, Millar LK, Koonings PP, Montoro M, Mestman JH. Perinatal outcome in hypothyroid pregnancies. *Obstet Gynecol*. 1993;81:349-53.
7. Haddow JE, Palomaki GE, Allan WC, Williams JR, Knight GJ, Gagnon J, et al. Maternal thyroid deficiency during pregnancy and subsequent neuropsychological development of the child. *N Engl J Med*. 1999;341:549-55.
8. Geenen V, Perrier de Hauterive S, Puit M, Hazout A, Goffin F, Frankenne F, et al. Autoimmunity and Pregnancy: theory and practice. *Acta Clin Belg*. 2002;57:317-24.
9. Thangaratinam S, Tan A, Knox E, Kilby MD, Franklyn J, Coomarasamy A. Association between thyroid autoantibodies and miscarriage and preterm birth: meta-analysis of evidence. *BMJ*. 2011;342:d2616.
10. Glinoer D. Management of hypo- and hyperthyroidism during pregnancy. *Growth Horm IGF Res*. 2003;13:S45-54.
11. Negro R, Formoso G, Mangieri T, Pezzarossa A, Dazzi D, Hassan H. Levothyroxine treatment in euthyroid pregnant women with autoimmune thyroid disease: Effects on obstetrical complications. *J Clin Endocrinol Metab*. 2006;91:2587-91.
12. Brent GA. Maternal thyroid function: interpretation of thyroid function tests in pregnancy. *Clin Obstet Gynecol*. 1997;40:3-15.
13. Alexander EK, Marqusee E, Lawrence J, Jarolim P, Fischer GA, Larsen PR. Timing and magnitude of increases in levothyroxine requirements during pregnancy in women with hypothyroidism. *N Engl J Med*. 2004;351:241-9.
14. Toft A. Increased levothyroxine requirements in pregnancy—Why, when, and how much? *N Engl J Med*. 2004;351:292-4.
15. Bungard TJ, Hurlburt M. Management of hypothyroidism during pregnancy. *CMAJ*. 2007;176:1077-8.
16. Stagnaro-Green A, Abalovich M, Alexander E, Azizi F, Mestman J, Negro R, et al. Guidelines of American Thyroid Association for Diagnosis and management of Thyroid Disease during pregnancy and postpartum. *Thyroid*. 2011;21:1081-125.

17. Guidelines for Management of Thyroid Dysfunction During Pregnancy. An Initiative from Indian Thyroid Society. Endorsed by- Endocrine Society of India. 2012. p. 5-6.
18. Vaidya B, Anthony S, Bilous M, Shields B, Drury J, Hutchison S, et al. Detection of thyroid dysfunction in early pregnancy: Universal screening or targeted high-risk case finding? *J Clin Endocrinol Metab.* 2007;92:203-7.
19. Muller AF, Drexhage HA, Berghout A. Postpartum thyroiditis and autoimmune thyroiditis in women of childbearing age: recent insights and consequences for antenatal and postnatal care. *Endocr Rev.* 2001;22:605-30.
20. Lucas A, Pizarro E, Granada ML, Salinas I, Roca J, Sanmartí A. Postpartum thyroiditis: long-term follow-up. *Thyroid.* 2005;15:1177-81.
21. Roti E, Emerson CH. Clinical review 29: Postpartum thyroiditis. *J Clin Endocrinol Metab.* 1992;74:3-5.

5

Thyrotoxicosis in Pregnancy

Sudeep K, Jubbin J Jacob

INTRODUCTION

Pregnancy is a temporary phase in women's reproductive life and is associated with unique physiological changes. The hormonal milieu of pregnancy alters the structural and functional profile of the thyroid gland. About 1–2% of women in the reproductive age group are affected by thyroid-related disorders, mainly hypothyroidism.[1] Hyperthyroidism is known to complicate only 1–2 women in 1000 pregnancies. Graves' disease, although rare in pregnancy, is, however, the most common cause of hyperthyroidism in pregnancy.[2] Both the disease and its therapy can affect the outcome in pregnancy.

MATERNAL THYROID PHYSIOLOGY IN PREGNANCY

The normal thyroid gland undergoes structural, hormonal/metabolic, and immunologic changes during pregnancy (Table 5-1), which are physiological adaptations to meet the dynamic demands of this phase. Some of these changes mimic thyrotoxicosis and are discussed in detail in the chapter, Endocrine Physiology in Pregnancy.

FETAL THYROID PHYSIOLOGY

During the first trimester, maternal thyroxine (T_4) is the only source of T_4 to the fetus. As shown in figure 5-1, maternal iodine, T_4, and thyroid antibodies cross the placenta while thyroid-stimulating hormone (TSH) does not.[3] The fetal thyroid gland becomes functional by the end of first trimester with iodide trapping and starts responding to TSH stimulation by 20th week.

TABLE 5-1

Thyroid-related Changes in Pregnancy	
Pregnancy-induced[4] physiological changes	*Consequent changes in thyroid functions*
Increased serum estrogen levels	Increase in serum TBG → binding of more T_4 and T_3 → less available free hormones stimulating more T_4 and T_3 output from the thyroid gland
Raised hCG	Reduced TSH and raised free T_4 (usually in reference range in most patients; beyond range in case of very high hCG levels)
Raised iodine clearance	Increased demand for iodine → increased gland size

TBG, thyroxine-binding globulin; T_4, thyroxine; T_3, triiodothryonine; TSH, thyroid-stimulating hormone; hCG, human chorionic gonadotropin.

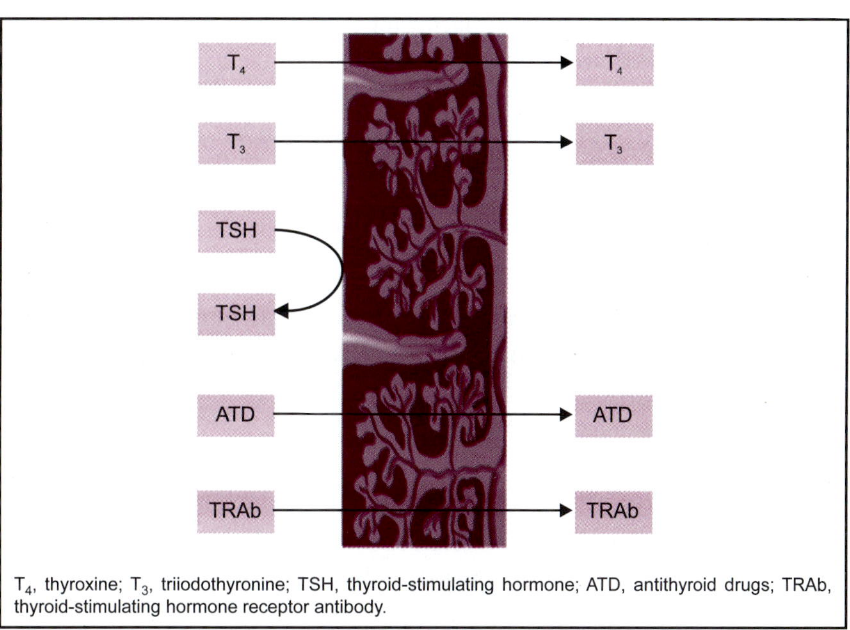

Figure 5-1 Placental transport of thyroid hormones, antithyroid drugs, and antibodies.

THYROID AUTOIMMUNITY IN PREGNANCY

During pregnancy, modulation in the immune system favors an environment that sustains the fetus without rejection. Hormonal changes induce both maternal and placental immune suppression. There is a reversible tilt favoring type 2 T helper (Th2) cells for type 1 T helper (Th1) cells, thus, attenuating the immune responsiveness during pregnancy.[4] This change is attributed to the increased progesterone-to-estrogen ratio. A rebound activation of autoimmune diseases is seen in the postpartum, as the immunosuppression of pregnancy weans off. Fetal microchimerism (fetal cells in maternal circulation) has been proposed to be one of the mechanisms of enhanced autoimmunity and manifestation of thyrotoxicosis in some individuals, inspite of the immunosuppression during pregnancy. Abnormalities in the inactivation or structure of the X-chromosome contribute to the impaired immune tolerance. The X-chromosome carries genes, which determine the sex hormone levels and also mediate immune tolerance. Disturbances in the inactivation of X-chromosome impair the thymic deletion of autoimmune cells.[4]

Risk Factors for Enhanced Thyroid Autoimmunity

Genetic

A higher incidence (16-fold) of autoimmune disorders in families has confirmed genetic susceptibility as an important factor for thyroid autoimmunity.[4] The cytotoxic T-lymphocyte-associated protein-4 (CTLA-4) is one of the confirmed major loci for thyroid autoimmunity. CD40 gene, protein tyrosine phosphatase-22 (PTPN22) gene, and CD25 gene are the other proposed genes shown to be associated with thyroid autoimmunity.

Other Factors

Iodine supplementation (enhances thyroid autoimmunity by expressing hidden genes), smoking, stress, environmental toxins, infections, and immune-modulating drugs are other risk factors, which can aggravate thyroid autoimmunity during pregnancy.

GRAVES' DISEASE

Graves' disease occurs in 1% of all females in the reproductive age group and is the most common cause (Table 5-2) of pregnancy hyperthyroidism (85–90%), occurring in 0.1–0.4% of pregnant women. It follows a triphasic course during pregnancy. Both antithyroid peroxidase (anti-TPO, in 60–90%) and TSH receptor antibody (TRAb, in 80–90%) are positive in Graves' disease, of which TRAb is more specific.

Effect of Pregnancy on Graves' Disease

Immunosuppression of pregnancy tends to prevent the development or resurgence of Graves' disease. Depending on the titer of the stimulating antibodies, hyperthyroidism can still occur or continue from the prepregnancy period to the first trimester. As pregnancy progresses, the disease severity wanes down significantly in parallel to the regressing antibody titers. It frequently relapses within 4–8 months after delivery.

TABLE 5-2

Causes of Thyrotoxicosis in Pregnancy	
Causes	*Remarks*
Common	
Graves' disease	Most common (85–90%)
Exogenous T_3 or T_4	History of drug intake
Iodine-induced hyperthyroidism	Long-standing goiter in endemic areas
Subacute thyroiditis	More significant in the postpartum period
Pregnancy-associated conditions	
Hyperemesis gravidarum	Transient, usually self-limiting as pregnancy progresses
Hydatidiform mole and other trophoblastic diseases of pregnancy	Reversible after evacuation of the mole
Rare	
Toxic multinodular goiter	Pregnancy occurs when they are mild or well controlled
Toxic adenoma	

T_3, triiodothyronine; T_4, thyroxine.

Effect of Graves' Disease on Pregnancy and Fetus

There are increased risks of miscarriage, preterm labor, stillbirths, and neonatal deaths in mothers with untreated or inadequately controlled Graves' disease.[5] They are more prone to preeclampsia, placental abruption, and cardiac failure when compared to those without toxicosis. Intrauterine exposure to high T_4 levels results in fetal tachycardia (heart rate >160/min), fetal hydrops, congestive cardiac failure, low birth weight, accelerated skeletal growth, goiter, growth retardation, and fetal malformations.[6] Neonatal hyperthyroidism is uncommon and is seen in less than 5% of the neonates born to thyrotoxic mothers. It is usually transient and lasts for a few weeks as the half-life of the thyroid antibodies is 3 weeks. It is due to the transplacental passage of maternal thyroid hormones and TRAb, which stimulates the fetal thyroid gland to produce goitre and excess T_4 production. Due to variability in the recovery of their hypothalamic-pituitary-thyroid axis, neonates born to mothers with severe thyrotoxicosis can even present with central hypothyroidism.[7] This necessitates monitoring of such infants for a longer period.

POSTPARTUM THYROIDITIS

This is due to the rebound autoimmune activity seen in 40–60% of those who are positive for anti-TPO antibodies. This can present as isolated thyrotoxicosis or a combined hyperthyroid phase followed by hypothyroid phase in the same individual or as an isolated hypothyroidism. This can occur even up to a year following delivery. Hyperthyroidism is usually transient and only requires symptomatic therapy with β-blockers. However, it has to be differentiated from reactivated Graves' disease where antithyroid drug therapy has to be initiated.

GESTATIONAL THYROTOXICOSIS

This biochemical abnormality, which is not antibody-mediated is seen in the first trimester when the human chorionic gonadotropin (hCG) levels peak at 10 weeks. TSH is in the lower limit of normal or is suppressed. The T_4 and triiodothyronine (T_3) levels are raised while the free T_4 levels may be in the upper limit of normal or just above it. Clinical correlation is often not seen, and as many as 50% of women may have symptoms like weight loss, tachycardia, etc. that overlap with an otherwise normal pregnancy. In those who do not have symptoms or goiter or eye signs, close follow-up is required as this normalizes spontaneously.

In hyperemesis gravidarum, hCG levels are higher than usual and the clinical features are more prominent. It presents with severe vomiting and ketonuria beginning at around 6–10 weeks and usually resolves spontaneously by 16–20 weeks. They sometimes require hospital admission for nutritional management. A biochemically overt disease with nonspecific signs of thyrotoxicosis is seen in about 50% of pregnant women having hyperemesis. The severity of hyperemesis and the thyroid activity correlates with the hCG levels.[8]

Gestational trophoblastic disease (both benign hydatidiform mole and malignant choriocarcinomas) has hCG levels that are 1000 folds higher than normal pregnancy. The serum T_4:T_3 ratio is much higher and clinical symptoms are more severe than in Graves' disease in spite of the minimal thyroid enlargement. Complete reversal of thyrotoxicosis occurs after removal of the mole.

Diagnosis

The diagnosis of thyrotoxicosis in pregnancy is complicated by the presence of overlapping clinical and biochemical features with normal pregnancy. Total T_3 and T_4 levels are normally up to 1.5 times higher than the nonpregnant reference range. Free T_4 is a better representative of the actual thyroid status, but its levels vary during each trimester of pregnancy. Automated analog-based assays for free T_4 and free T_3 estimation differ between manufacturers. It is recommended to have a method-specific reference range for the 3 trimesters from each manufacturer.

A diagnosis of thyrotoxicosis is considered when we have elevated thyroid hormone levels above the pregnancy range and a suppressed (<0.1) or undetectable TSH (<0.01).

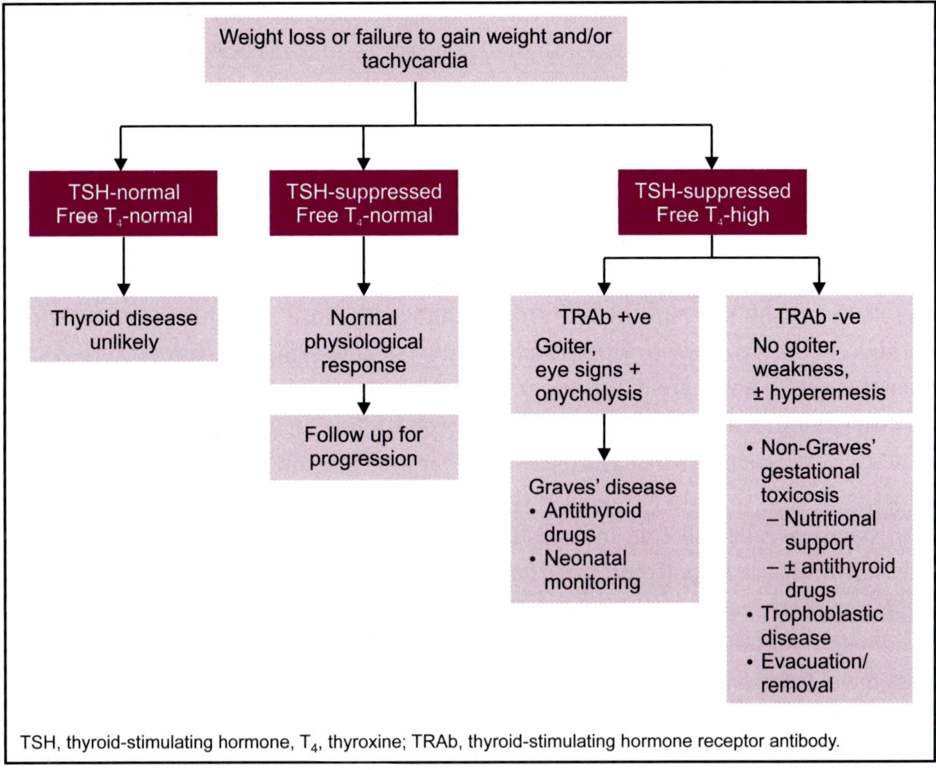

Figure 5-2 Work-up of a patient with suspected hyperthyroidism during pregnancy.

In such situations, the presence of diffuse goiter, eye signs, and a high TRAb titer confirms Graves' disease. In the absence of these features, an elevated free T_4 just above the reference range with tachycardia and weight loss should be carefully interpreted (Figure 5-2). Even when overt biochemical thyrotoxicosis is present, differentiating a transient phenomenon from that of Graves' disease is vital, as the former seldom requires antithyroid drug therapy.

TRAb is a very good indicator of autoimmune thyroid activity and has 95% sensitivity and 99% specificity in establishing the diagnosis of Graves' disease. It also helps in predicting the risk of thyroid dysfunction in the fetus. In the second half of pregnancy, a high TRAb titer raises the possibility of neonatal hyperthyroidism, as these antibodies can cross the placenta. Conversely, a shift from TRAb-positive state to a TRAb-negative state during pregnancy is an indication for stopping antithyroid drug therapy, as there is a risk of neonatal hypothyroidism. In mothers who had prior thyroid ablation or thyroidectomy, antibodies are measured in the first trimester and, if positive, are measured again at the 22–26 weeks of gestation.[9] TRAb measurement also helps differentiate postpartum Graves' disease from postpartum thyroiditis. TRAb measurement is not required in antithyroid drug treated Graves' disease, who are in remission and have withdrawn antithyroid drugs prior to conception.

Management

Mild Graves' disease may regress spontaneously as pregnancy progresses. These patients do not require antithyroid drug therapy and this usually is seen in mothers whose TRAb titers are negative or low. Moderate-to-severe Graves' disease needs antithyroid drug therapy.[10] In patients in whom an occult Graves' disease cannot be ruled out but have severe symptoms, antithyroid drug therapy with close monitoring can be tried. Antithyroid drug therapy is withdrawn once the patient's symptoms have reversed and when the free T_4 levels are in the upper limit of normal.

Propylthiouracil (PTU) is the treatment of choice particularly during the first trimester of pregnancy. Methimazole (MMI)/carbimazole can be initiated after the first trimester or if PTU is not available or the patient does not tolerate PTU.[11] Antithyroid drug therapy is relatively safe and is usually associated with minor side effects like skin rashes, arthralgia, and gastrointestinal disturbances that occur only in a subset of patients. Major and life threatening side effects like agranulocytosis (0.35–0.45%), polyarthritis, vasculitis, and immunoallergic hepatitis can occur rarely. Like TRAb, antithyroid drugs cross the placenta, and MMI has higher incidence of aplasia cutis and esophageal and choanal atresias when compared to PTU. Although relatively safe, PTU can cause vasculitis, antineutrophil cytoplasmic antibody positivity (40 times more than MMI), and a rare immunoallergic hepatotoxicity (0.1–0.2%). When patients with Graves' disease on MMI become pregnant, they should be switched over to PTU during the first trimester and can be switched back to MMI thereafter.[11] PTU is initiated at the dose of 100–150 mg every 8 hourly and then reduced to 50 mg thrice daily based on the T_4 and free T_4 levels. A 10–15 mg dose of MMI is roughly equivalent to 300 mg of PTU (i.e., 10–15:1). If PTU is being continued beyond the first trimester, liver enzymes should be monitored every month.

Maternal heart rate, weight gain, and goiter size are used for clinical assessment. Maternal thyroid hormone levels are measured every 2–4 weeks and the dose of antithyroid drugs is adjusted. The T_3, T_4, and free T_4 levels are maintained at the upper one-third or just above the trimester-specific reference range for pregnancy.[10] TSH is allowed to remain suppressed (0.1–0.4), and the dose is reduced when it starts to normalize. The lowest possible dose is used to avoid fetal hypothyroidism and/or goiter. While on antithyroid drugs, the fetus should be monitored for growth, development of goiter, and bradycardia. Once TSH levels reach the normal range, antithyroid drugs should be withdrawn. Antithyroid drug therapy has been shown to adequately control the toxic state with a favorable maternal and fetal outcome when properly monitored and utilized.[12] Some authors prefer continuing minimum dose of antithyroid drugs during the third trimester after achieving euthyroidism in order to prevent postpartum recurrence of Graves' disease.[13]

β-blockers may be used for a short duration to reduce the hypermetabolic symptoms or while waiting for surgery. It has to be kept in mind that they may cause intra-uterine growth retardation (IUGR) on prolonged usage and also carry a risk of fetal hypoglycemia and bradycardia, when used late in pregnancy.[12] Iodides are not used during pregnancy. Recommendations for the management of thyrotoxicosis during pregnancy by Indian Thyroid Society (ITS) have been tabulated in table 5-3.

Thyroid Surgery

When a pregnant mother is not responding to high dose of antithyroid drugs (>300 mg of PTU or 40 mg of carbimazole) or gets adverse reactions with antithyroid drugs, subtotal thyroidectomy is indicated. Because of the potential adverse effects of the anesthetic agents on the fetus and an increased risk of pregnancy loss, thyroidectomy is avoided in the first trimester. The second trimester is optimal for thyroidectomy, but it still carries a 4.5–5% risk of preterm labor. Preoperative preparation with iodine is carried out 1–2 weeks prior to surgery to reduce the gland vascularity and hormone release.

OTHER DISORDERS

Majority of women with gestational thyrotoxicosis require follow-up. In case of hyperemesis (those presenting with ketonuria, weight loss of >5%, and dehydration), the mothers should be evaluated for thyroid dysfunction. Rarely, some of them with overt toxicosis may require antithyroid drugs for a short duration. Otherwise, they require conservative management with parenteral nutrition till the hyperemesis subsides. The ITS guidelines recommend thyroid function tests to be done in all patients with hyperemesis.[14] It also recommends considering antithyroid drugs only in those exceptional cases where the thyroid functions are persistently abnormal beyond 18–20 weeks of pregnancy.

Treatment of subclinical thyrotoxicosis is not recommended as there is no evidence to show that the outcome improves. Treating with antithyroid drugs may potentially produce adverse outcomes because the presence of T_3 and T_4 levels at or just above the reference ranges is actually beneficial.

When there is a suspicion of pregnancy or if there is confirmed pregnancy, radioiodine (I-131) should not be given. If inadvertently treated, the patient should be promptly informed of the adverse effects of radiation to the fetus, including thyroid destruction, if treated after the 12th week of gestation. There is no data, for or against, recommending termination of pregnancy after I-131 exposure.

TABLE 5-3

Recommendations of ITS for Management of Thyrotoxicosis During Pregnancy
• Hyperthyroidism should be distinguished from normal physiological thyroid functions during pregnancy and hyperemesis gravidarum in case of subnormal serum TSH during pregnancy. Presence of TRAb and diffuse goiter are evident in the diagnosis of Graves' disease
• In case of overt hyperthyroidism diagnosed during pregnancy, PTU is the drug of choice, especially in the first trimester and should be started immediately. In case of intolerance of PTU by the patient, MMI/carbimazole should be substituted
• Due to the adverse effects caused by long-term use of β-blockers, they should be recommended only for symptomatic control of thyrotoxicosis or while awaiting response to the antithyroid medications or surgery. Propranolol is the most commonly used β-blocker
• Iodides can lead to fetal goiter and should not be used
• When antithyroid drugs fail to control the hyperthyroid disease (over 300 mg/day of PTU or 40 mg/day MMI/carbimazole), surgery is indicated. Second trimester is the safest time suggested for surgery
• During pregnancy, use of I-131 is contraindicated because of the possible teratogenic effects of radiation. Effective contraception is recommended for at least 3 months following therapy. There are no data, for or against, recommending termination of pregnancy after inadvertent exposure of I-131
• If pregnancy occurs in active Graves' disease, treatment with an antithyroid drug should be continued. TRAb titers could be assessed in third trimester, if possible, to determine if the fetus is at risk of developing hyperthyroidism
• If a relapse occurs in a woman with a previous history of Graves' disease during early pregnancy, medication should be restarted
• In case of pregnancy after a previous ablative treatment, reassessment of TRAb levels (if possible) at the beginning of pregnancy is recommended to determine the chance of fetal or postnatal hyper- or hypothyroidism
• If the mother is euthyroid but positive for TRAb, a possibility of fetal thyrotoxicosis arises that should be assessed by FHR (>160 bpm). If all other causes of fetal tachycardia have been ruled out, MMI/carbimazole should be given to mother in order to control fetal thyrotoxicosis and LT_4 to maintain maternal euthyroidism
• Pregnant women with TRAb or those treated with antithyroid drugs should have a fetal ultrasound to detect fetal thyroid dysfunction. This may include growth restriction, hydrops, presence of goiter, and cardiac failure
• Once fetal hyperthyroidism is diagnosed, antithyroid drug therapy should be administered to the mother. The fetus should be re-evaluated for clinical improvement (heart rate, goiter resolution) by ultrasound in 2 weeks and appropriate dose adjustment should be done
• Umbilical blood sampling should be considered only, if the diagnosis of fetal thyroid disease is not reasonably certain from the clinical data and, if the information gained would change the treatment
• Presence of subclinical hyperthyroidism (normal serum fetal T_4 levels and a low serum TSH level) in pregnant women does not warrant any treatment.

ITS, Indian Thyroid Society; PTU, propylthiouracil; T_4, thyroxine; TRAb, thyroid-stimulating hormone receptor antibody; TSH, thyroid-stimulating hormone; I-131, radioiodine; FHR, fetal heart rate; MMI, methimazole.

Source: Guidelines for Management of Thyroid Dysfunction During Pregnancy. An Initiative from Indian Thyroid Society. Endorsed by- Endocrine Society of India. 2012; *with permission.*

Euthyroid or hypothyroid mothers who had radioiodine ablation and thyroid surgery for Graves' disease prior to their pregnancy carry a risk of fetal thyroid dysfunction, as they have persistent TRAb production because of the absence of antithyroid drugs. Fetal ultrasound should be performed at 28–32 weeks to look for evidences of fetal thyroid dysfunction like diffuse doppler signals in the fetal thyroid.[15] The presence of fetal tachycardia (>160/min) is an indication for the initiation of antithyroid drugs to control fetal hyperthyroidism along with thyroxine to maintain maternal euthyroidism. Sonographic monitoring of the fetus should be continued for assessing the response and adjusting the antithyroid drugs. Umbilical blood sampling is restricted to those instances where clinical information is not certain or only if the information gained by doing so can change the outcome.

All neonates born to thyrotoxic mothers should be screened for thyroid dysfunction and may require repeat tests after few days.[7] Antithyroid drug therapy and β-blockers are initiated with MMI (0.5–1 mg/kg) or PTU (5–10 mg/kg) in neonates with hyperthyroidism. Propranolol is given in the dose of 2 mg/kg. In case of severe thyrotoxicosis, glucocorticoids or oral iodine solutions can be used.[12]

During lactation, reactivated Graves' disease can be treated with antithyroid drugs, particularly MMI, as there is a risk of hepatotoxicity with PTU. Antithyroid drugs are safe for infants being breastfed by their thyrotoxic mothers.[16] A total daily dose of 20 mg MMI and 450 mg PTU taken after a breastfeed by the mother has been found to be safe by Mandel et al.[17]

During the postpartum, high-risk mothers should be monitored for resurgence of Graves' disease or postpartum thyroiditis. Mothers who had Graves' disease and had entered remission during pregnancy, those with type 1 diabetes, or who had TPO positivity in first trimester should have their thyroid functions assessed in the third and sixth months postpartum, as they have a significant risk for relapse of Graves' disease or postpartum thyroiditis.[14,17]

THYROID STORM

It is the most severe form of thyrotoxicosis usually affecting only a fraction (1–2%) of thyrotoxic patients. It is rare in pregnancy and is precipitated by infection, surgery, preeclampsia, and labor. It is characterized by severe features of toxicosis with fever and altered mentation. Treatment of the precipitating causes like infection along with aggressive treatment of the toxicosis is very important. In addition to antithyroid drugs, β-blockers, iodide, and glucocorticoids (dexamethasone to inhibit the peripheral conversion of T_4 to T_3) are used along with temperature lowering measures. Fluid and electrolytes should be managed appropriately along with close fetal monitoring. PTU that has an additional advantage of inhibiting peripheral conversion of T_4 to T_3 is preferred over MMI. Iodide is given at least 1 hour after starting PTU therapy.

Medications are given through nasogastric tube or as rectal suppositories. Subsequent definitive treatment, either thyroidectomy or radioiodine ablation, should be planned prior to the next pregnancy.

CONCLUSION

Thyrotoxicosis during pregnancy, although uncommon, is associated with diagnostic and therapeutic difficulties. Gestational thyrotoxicosis and hyperemesis of pregnancy may mimic Graves' disease. Antithyroid drug therapy is used as the first-line therapy in moderate-to-severe Graves' disease. PTU is given in the first trimester and thereafter can be switched over to MMI. In situations where antithyroid drugs cannot be continued, thyroidectomy is performed, preferably in the second trimester. TRAb assessment helps in certain situations. Newborn cord blood TSH and free T_4 should be measured in situations where the mother has a high risk for transplacental passage of antithyroid drugs or TRAb. Antithyroid drug therapy is safe during lactation.

REFERENCES

1. Burrow GN. Thyroid function and hyperfunction during gestation. *Endocr Rev*. 1993;14: 194-202.
2. Mestman JH. Hyperthyroidism in pregnancy. *Endocrinol Metab Clin North Am*. 1998;27: 127-49.
3. Chan GW, Mandel SJ. Therapy Insight: management of Graves' disease during pregnancy. *Nat Clin Pract Endocrinol Metab*. 2007;3:470-8.
4. Gaberšček S, Zaletel K. Thyroid physiology and autoimmunity in pregnancy and after delivery. *Expert Rev Clin Immunol*. 2011;7:697-707.
5. Millar LK, Wing DA, Leung AS, Koonings PP, Montoro MN, Mestman JH. Low birth weight and preeclampsia in pregnancies complicated by hyperthyroidism. *Obstet Gynecol*. 1994;84:946-9.
6. Mitsuda N, Tamaki H, Amino N, Hosono T, Miyai K, Tanizawa O. Risk factors for developmental disorders in infants born to women with Graves' disease. *Obstet Gynecol*. 1992;80:359-64.
7. Sarathi HA, Bandgar T, Shah NS. Delayed recognition of central hypothyroidism in a neonate born to thyrotoxic mother. *Indian Pediatr*. 2010;47:795-6.
8. Fantz CR, Dagogo S, Ladenson JH, Gronowski AM. Thyroid Function during Pregnancy. *Clin Chem*. 1999;45:2250-8.
9. Vos XG, Smit N, Endert E, Tijssen JG, Wiersingha WM. Frequency and characteristics of TBII seronegative patients in a population with untreated Graves' hyperthyroidism: a prospective study. *Clin Endocrinol (Oxf)*. 2008;69:311-7.
10. Momotani N, Noh J, Oyanagi H, Ishikawa N, Ito K. Antithyroid drug therapy for Graves' disease during pregnancy. Optimal regimen for fetal thyroid status. *N Engl J Med*. 1986; 315:24-8.

11. The Endocrine Society. Management of thyroid dysfunction during pregnancy and postpartum: an Endocrine Society clinical practice guideline. Chevy Chase (MD): The Endocrine Society; 2007. p. 79.
12. Dwarakanath CS, Ammini AC, Kriplani A, Shah P, Paul VK. Graves' Disease during pregnancy—results of antithyroid drug therapy. *Singapore Med J*. 1999;40:70-3.
13. Azizi F, Amouzegar A. Management of hyperthyroidism during pregnancy and lactation. *Eur J Endocrinol*. 2011;164:871-6.
14. Guidelines for Management of Thyroid Dysfunction During Pregnancy. An Initiative from Indian Thyroid Society. Endorsed by- Endocrine Society of India. 2012. p. 12-4.
15. Luton D, Le Gac I, Vuillard E, Castanet M, Guibourdenche J, Noel M, et al. Management of Graves' disease during pregnancy: the key role of fetal thyroid gland monitoring. *J Clin Endocrinol Metab*. 2005;90:6093-8.
16. Azizi F, Khoshniat M, Bahrainian M, Hedayati M. Thyroid function and intellectual development of infants nursed by mothers taking methimazole. *J Clin Endocrinol Metab*. 2000;85:3233-8.
17. Mandel SJ, Cooper DS. The use of antithyroid drugs in pregnancy and lactation. *J Clin Endocrinol Metab*. 2001;86:2354-9.
18. Rotondi M, Cappelli C, Pirali B, Pirola I, Magri F, Fonte R, et al. The effect of pregnancy on subsequent relapse from Graves' disease after a successful course of antithyroid drug therapy. *J Clin Endocrinol Metab*. 2008;93:3985-8.

6

Parathyroid Disorders During Pregnancy

Rajesh Rajput

INTRODUCTION

The disorders of parathyroid gland are not only uncommon in pregnant women, but their recognition is also difficult during pregnancy, because of lack of specific symptoms and satisfactory physical examination. However, if unrecognized, they may result in significant perinatal and maternal morbidity and mortality. Improved understanding, better diagnostic studies, and efficient management decisions can significantly improve the outcomes in mothers and their unborn children.

CALCIUM METABOLISM DURING PREGNANCY

The developing fetus needs about 30 g of calcium for skeletal growth, and majority of it (approximately, 80%) is needed during the third trimester. To meet this fetal demand of calcium and the state of hypercalciuria normally present in pregnancy, many physiological adaptations take place in the body of pregnant women.[1]

Since total calcium levels are decreased during pregnancy due to physiological hypoalbuminemia, the upper limit of normal values for total serum calcium is 9.5 mg/dL. The ionized calcium levels remain normal during pregnancy. The serum levels of 25-hydroxy vitamin D [25(OH)D] remain unchanged during pregnancy, but due to estrogen-induced increase in vitamin D binding globulin and increase in 1-α hydoxylase activity secondary to rising estrogen and human placental lactogen (HPL) levels, there is twofold rise in 1,25-dihydroxy vitamin D3 [$1,25(OH)_2D3$] levels after the first trimester. The increase in this active vitamin-D metabolite, i.e., $1,25(OH)_2D3$ results in enhanced calcium absorption from gut during pregnancy (Figure 6-1). There is also an increased synthesis of calcitonin, which opposes $1,25(OH)_2D3$ to absorb calcium from bones, so that calcium is provided to the developing fetus from maternal gut rather than maternal skeleton. In pregnant

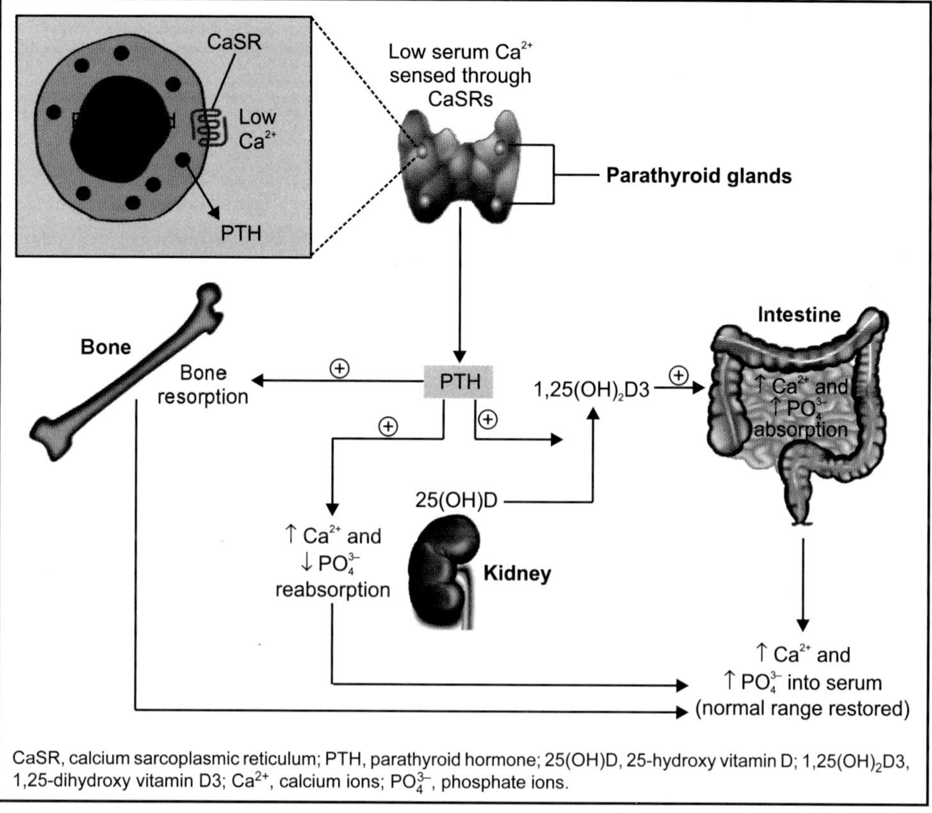

CaSR, calcium sarcoplasmic reticulum; PTH, parathyroid hormone; 25(OH)D, 25-hydroxy vitamin D; $1,25(OH)_2D3$, 1,25-dihydroxy vitamin D3; Ca^{2+}, calcium ions; PO_4^{3-}, phosphate ions.

Figure 6-1 Calcium metabolism during pregnancy.

women, despite an increase in total parathyroid hormone (PTH), the concentration of its intact form is either normal or reduced. The fall in PTH probably is a physiological response to increased parathyroid hormone-related protein (PTHrP) levels, which is presumably derived from placenta and mammary gland or fetal parathyroid gland. The placental transport of calcium is stimulated by PTHrP (1-141) and midmolecule of PTHrP (67-86) but not by PTH (1-34) during pregnancy.[1-3]

After delivery, significant changes occur in calcium metabolism when compared to pregnancy. The urinary calcium excretion reduces, concenteration of $1,25(OH)_2D3$ and PTH returns to prepregnancy levels, but PTHrP levels remain elevated for promoting transfer of calcium across breast tissue.[2]

The ionized calcium levels are higher in the cord blood than in normal adults and when placenta is removed, the calcium levels fall to 4–4.7 mg/dL within 1–2 days after birth. Plasma PTH levels are also low in neonates, and they are minimally responsive to low calcium levels for first 2–3 days of life, leading to transient neonatal hypocalcemia. In infants born to mothers with primary hyperparathyroidism (PHPT), there is a high incidence of symptomatic hypocalcemia due to suppression of prenatal parathyroid development during the entire pregnancy.[4]

PRIMARY HYPERPARATHYROIDISM

The first case of PHPT in pregnancy was reported in 1931.[5] The incidence of PHPT in women of childbearing age is around 8 new cases per 100,000 population per year.[6,7] It is presumed that a lack of recognition or under reporting during pregnancy is responsible for an apparently lower incidence, as majority of women are asymptomatic during pregnancy and those with mild symptoms are misdiagnosed of having these as secondary to physiological changes during pregnancy. The degree of hypercalcemia is masked by increased demands of the developing fetus along with increased maternal clearance and physiological hypoalbuminemia during pregnancy. Pregnancy seems to protect the patients from developing the sequelae of PHPT, which may decrease the likelihood of subsequent diagnosis.[3]

Although PHPT does not affect fertility in women, it increases chances of stillbirth or spontaneous abortion. The most common pathology of PHPT in nonpregnant patients is a single parathyroid adenoma accounting for about 80% of cases. Hyperplasia of all the four glands was seen in 15% of cases reported, 3% of patients had adenoma in multiple glands, and a parathyroid carcinoma was detected in 2% of cases.[8]

Maternal Complications

Various studies indicate that the maternal complication rate in PHPT can be as high as 67%.[9] Pregnancy is a state of increased absorptive hypercalciuria. This along with increased calcium from PHPT can result in nephrolithiasis. There is also an increased incidence of urinary tact infections and pyelonephritis, presumably due to increased incidence of nephrocalcinosis and nephrolithiasis. The incidence of nephrolithiasis during pregnancy is 24–36% as compared to 20% during nonpregnant state. Radiograhic bone disease is seen in 13–19% of pregnant patients (24% in nonpregnant patients).[10,11] Pancreatitis, which complicates hyperparathyroidism in 1–2% of the general population, poses a greater risk in pregnancy with a 7–13% reported prevalence. It is more common in primipara than in multipara, in first and third trimesters, and postpartum.[12,13] The risk of hyperemesis gravidarum inceases in pregnancy with PHPT. One of the most feared complication of PHPT is hypercalcemic crisis. This condition rarely occurs during gestation and presents classically with hypercalcemia (usually >14 mg/dL), nausea, vomiting, weakness, dehydration, and mental status changes, which can rapidly progress to uremia, coma, and death.[13] Women who are not identified and adequately treated during pregnancy can have worsening of hypercalcemia after delivery, as the protective effects of fetus and placenta are lost.

Fetal Complications

The incidence of fetal complications in untreated patients is around 80%. Even in conservatively treated patients, the incidence of complications is around 53%. Various complications include intrauterine growth retardation (IUGR), low birth weight, preterm delivery, and even intrauterine fetal death. Neonatal hypocalcemia develops between 2 and 14 days of life and lasts for few days. The severity of hypocalcemia is related to maternal serum calcium levels, with 50% of neonates born to untreated mothers developing tetany later. Although it is usually transient, it can persist for few months and several cases of permanent neonatal hypocalcemia have been reported.[14]

Diagnosis

A high index of suspicion in any pregnant woman with serum calcium more than 9.5 mg/dL is needed for making a diagnosis of PHPT during pregnancy. The diagnosis of PHPT is based on persistent hypercalcemia in presence of an increased serum PTH levels. In few patients, serum PTH levels may be in the upper limit of normal range but inappropriate for the degree of hypercalcemia. 24-hour urinary calcium excretion is also increased in comparison to that seen in normal pregnancy. Ultrasound of neck can be done to locate parathyroid adenomas in suspicious cases. The sensitivity and specificity of ultrasound is 67% and 94%, respectively.[15] Alternatively, the risk benefit ratio of computed tomography (CT) or magnetic resonance imaging (MRI) should be considered, which may identify lesions missed with ultrasound. Radionuclide sestamibi scan is not indicated for localization of parathyroid adenoma during pregnancy.

Differential Diagnosis of Hypercalcemia During Pregnancy

Although hypercalcemia during pregnancy can be due to many causes as seen in nonpregnant women, three uncommon syndromes associated with hypercalcemia during pregnancy include familial hypocalciuric hypercalcemia (FHH), postpartum hypercalcemia in women treated for hypoparathyroidism, and PTHrP related hypercalcemia.

FHH is an autosomal dominant condition caused by inactivating mutation in the gene for calcium sensing receptor in kidney and parathyroid gland. Patients usually present with mild hypercalcemia, mild hypermagnesemia, low urinary calcium excretion, and mild elevation in PTH levels along with moderate enlargement of the 4 parathyroid glands. Asymptomatic hypercalcemia (neonate is a carrier), severe neonatal hypocalcemia, and severe neonatal hypercalcemia (infant homozygous for mutated gene) requiring parathyroidectomy, can be the presenting clinical manifestations in neonates.[16]

Postpartum hypercalcemia develops in women treated with vitamin D and calcium during pregnancy for hypoparathyroidism. The exact mechanism for these changes is not well understood. Patients present with nausea and vomiting few days after delivery, and calcium and vitamin D need to be discontinued in such cases.[17]

PTHrP related hypercalcemia has been described during pregnancy and postpartum period. Khosla et al. reported a patient with bilateral breast enlargement and serum calcium of 14.5 mg/dL and undetectable PTH. The patient underwent bilateral mastectomy, and her breast tissue showed PTHrP antigenic activity on immunohistochemistry.[18] Tarnawa et al. recently reported a patient with severe hypercalcemia associated with uterine leiomyoma during pregnancy. Her serum calcium was 15.9 mg/dL, PTH below 3 pg/mL, vitamin D 15 pg/mL, and PTHrP 22 pmol/L (normally <2).[19]

Management

The definitive treatment of PHPT is removal of abnormal parathyroid glands. This should preferably be done in the second trimester, although the risk benefit ratio favors surgical treatment even in third trimester. For asymptomatic women with calcium levels below 11 mg/dL, there is no sufficient evidence in literature on proper management; although surgical management appears to be reasonable because of increased complications with advancing pregnancy. Indications for parathyroidectomy are described in table 6-1.

Medical therapy in the form of oral phosphate is reserved for patients who are not surgical candidates. Side efects of oral phosphate are nausea, vomiting, and hypokalemia.[20] Use of bisphosphonates is not recommended during pregnancy. Good hydration, early treatment of urinary tract infection, and avoiding medications that may increase calcium levels like vitamin D, aminophylline, and thiazide diuretics are important therapeutic measures.

In patients undergoing surgery, serum calcium should be checked every 6 hours to detect postoperative hypocalcemia. Patients with severe bone disease are likely to develop hungry bone syndrome and profound hypocalcemia postoperatively. If symptomatic, it should be treated with intravenous calcium gluconate given at a rate of 0.5–2 mg/kg/hour along with calcitriol 0.5–1.0 μg/day.[21]

TABLE 6-1

Indications for Parathyroid Surgery in the Pregnant Women
• Symptomatic hyperparathyroidism
• Serum calcium >11 mg/dL
• History of life-threatning hypercalcemic crisis
• Reduction of age and pregnancy-matched creatinine clearance by more than 30% without another explanation
• Presence of nephrolithiasis/nephrocalcinosis and radiographic bone disease.

HYPOPARATHYROIDISM

Hypoparathyroidism is characterized by hypocalcemia and hyperphosphatemia. It usually presents with symptoms of hypocalcemia and include numbness and tingling of fingers, toes, and around lips. Convulsions may be manifestation of severe hypoparathyroidism. Patient may complain of carpopedal spasms, laryngeal stridor, or dyspnea, with bronchial asthma considered to be equivalent to tetany. Use of various tocolytics during pregnancy can exacerbate symptoms of hypoparathyroidism. Physical examination includes positive Chvostek's sign (twitch of facial muscle when a tap is given on facial nerve) and Trousseau's sign (carpopedal spasm by reducing circulation of arm by blood pressure cuff). In severe and long standing cases, papilledema, cataract, and ectopic calcification at various body sites may be seen. Persistent hypocalcemia is also dangerous for the developing fetus, as hypocalcaemia tends to increase uterine irritability which possibly may cause induction of preterm labor.[22]

The most common cause of hypoparathyroidism is removal or damage to parathyroid gland during thyroid surgery. The risk of hypoparathyroidism is 0.5–6.6% after thyroid surgery, which depends on baseline thyroid disorder, thyroid volume, percentage of thyroid ablation, and personal experience of the surgeon. Idiopathic hypoparathyroidism is another rare cause which is usually associated with autoimmune endocrinopathy and calcium sensing receptor mutation. The diagnosis is confirmed by low serum calcium levels and high phosphate levels with low PTH levels. Plasma alkaline phosphatase levels are normal.[23]

In the past, diagnosis of hypoparathyroidism during pregnancy was considered as an indication for elective abortion, which is not true nowadays. Treatment of hypoparathyroidism during pregnancy does not differ from that of nonpregnant state. Calcitriol [1,25$(OH)_2$D3] is the treatment of choice, as it has a short half-life and chances of toxicity are less as compared to alfacalcidiol (1 α-hydroxy cholecalciferol) that has a longer half-life. Normal calcium requirement during pregnancy is 1200–1500 mg/day. Calcitriol 0.25 μg/day and a calcium supplementation of 1 g/day should be initiated, and later the dose should be adjusted. The dosage of calcitriol and calcium needs to be increased after 20th week of gestation with further elevation in the last trimester. Serum calcium levels should not fall below 7.0 mg/dL (1.70 mmol/L) to avoid preterm labor or mid-trimester abortion. During lactation, calcitriol should be reduced with an aim of avoiding hypercalcemia in both mother and baby.[24]

CONCLUSION

Hypo- or hyperparathyroidism during pregnancy, although rare, can cause significant maternal as well as fetal complications. Most of the cases go undiagnosed during pregnancy due to lack of appropriate physical examination and specific symptomatology. The sequelae of the disease does not develop because of the protective mechanism provided by pregnancy. However, with misdiagnosis, the chances of abortion or stillbirth are heightened to a great degree. Prompt diagnosis and treatment of parathyroid disorders during pregnancy is, therefore, required to prevent maternal or fetal morbidity and mortality.

REFERENCES

1. Braunstein GD. Endocrine changes in pregnancy. In: Kronenberg HM, Melmed S, Polonsky KS, Larsen PR eds. William's Textbook of Endocrinology. 11th ed. Philadelphia, PA: Saunders; 2008. p. 741-54.
2. Hirota Y, Anai T, Miyakawa I. Parathyroid hormone related protein levels in maternal and cord blood. *Am J Obstet Gynecol.* 1997;177:702-6.
3. Pitkin RM. Calcium and the parathyroid gland. In: Burrows GN, Ferris TF eds.: Medical Complications during Pregnancy. 4th ed. Philadelphia, PA: Saunders; 1995. p. 210-7.
4. MacIsaac RJ, Heath JA, Rodda CP, Moseley JM, Care AD, Martin TJ, et al. Role of the fetal parathyroid glands and the parathyroid hormone related protein in the regulation of placental transport of calcium, magnesium and inorganic phosphate. *Reprod Fertil Dev.* 1991;3:447-57.
5. Hunter D, Turnbull HM. Hyperparathyroidism: Generalized osteitis fibrosa with observations upon bones, parathyroid tumors and the normal parathyroid glands. *Br J Surg.* 1931;19:203-6.
6. Wermers RA, Khosla S, Atkinson EJ, Hodgson SF, O'Fallen WM, Meltan LJ 3rd. The rise and fall of primary hyperparathyroidism: A population based study in Rochester, Minnesota, 1965–1992. *Ann Intern Med.* 1997;26:433-40.
7. Haenel LC 4th, Mayfield RK. Primary hyperparathyroidism in a twin pregnancy and review of fetal/maternal calcium homeostasis. *Am J Med Sci.* 2000;319:191-4.
8. Silverberg SJ, Bilezikina AE. Primary hyperparathyroidism. In: DeGrout LF, Jameson JL, Potts JT, eds. Endocrinology. 4th Ed. Philadelphia, PA: WB Saunders Co; 2001. p. 969-98.
9. Kort KC, Schiller HJ, Numann PJ. Hyperparathyroidism and pregnancy. *Am J Surg.* 1999; 177:66-8.
10. Silverberg SJ. Natural history of primary hyperparathyroidism. *Endocrinol Metab Clin North Am.* 2000;29:541-64.
11. Silverberg SJ, Shane E, Jacobs TP, Siris E, Bilezikion P. A 10-year prospective study of primary hyperparathyroidism with or without parathyroid surgery. *N Engl J Med.* 1999;341: 1249-55.
12. Fabrin B, Eldon K. Pregnancy complicated by concurrent hyperparathyroidism and pancreatitis. *Acta Obstet Gynecol Scand.* 1986;65:651-2.
13. Clark D, Seeds JW, Cefalo RC. Hyperparathyroid crisis and pregnancy. *Am J Obstet Gynecol.* 1981;140:840-2.
14. Kelly TR. Primary hyperparathyroidism during pregnancy. *Surgery.* 1991;110:1028-34.
15. Sauer M, Steere A, Parsons MT. Hyperparathyroidism in pregnancy with sonographic documentation of a parathyroid adenoma. A case report. *J Reprod Med.* 1985;30:615-7.

16. Pearce SH, Trump D, Wooding C, Besser GM, Chew SL, Grant DB, et al. Calcium sensing receptor mutation in familial benign hypercalcemia and neonatal hyperparathyroidism. *J Clin Invest.* 1995;96:2683-92.
17. Wright AD, Joplin GF, Dixon HG. Postpartum hypercalcemia in treated hypoparathyroidism. *BMJ.* 1969;1:23-5.
18. Khosla S, van Heerden JA, Gharib H, Jackson IT, Danks J, Hayman JA, et al. Parathyroid hormone related protein and hypercalcemia secondary to massive mammary hyperplasia. *N Engl J Med.* 1990;322:1157.
19. Tarnawa E, Sullivan S, Underwood P, Richardson M, Spruill L. Severe Hypercalcemia Associated With Uterine Leiomyoma in Pregnancy. *Obstet Gynecol.* 2011;117:473-6.
20. Levy HA, Pierucci L, Stroup P. Oral phosphates treatment Primary Hyperparathyroidism in Pregnancy. *J Med Soc N J.* 1981;78:113-5.
21. Trupka A, Hallfeldt K, Horn K, Gartner R, Landgraf R. Intraoperative monitoring of intact parathyroid hormone (iPTH) in surgery of primary hyperparathyroidism with a new rapid test. *Chirurg.* 2001;72:578-83.
22. Shoback D. Clinical practice. Hypoparathyroidism. *N Engl J Med.* 2008;359:391-403.
23. Graham WP 3rd, Gordon GS, Loken HF, Blum A, Halden A. Effect of pregnancy and of the menstrual cycle on hypoparathyroidism. *J Clin Endocrinol Metab.* 1964;24:512-6.
24. Salle BL, Berthezene F, Glorieux GH, Delvin EE, Berland M, David L, et al. Hypoparathyroidism during pregnancy: treatment with calcitriol. *J Clin Endocrinol Metab.* 1981;52:810-3.

7

Endocrinology of Hyperemesis Gravidarum

Roopa Verghese, Jewel Jacob, Jubbin J Jacob

INTRODUCTION

Nausea and vomiting in pregnancy is extremely common. It occurs in over 50–90% of all pregnancies. It usually begins by 9–10 weeks of gestation, peaks at 11–13 weeks, and resolves in most cases by 12–14 weeks. In about 1–10% of pregnancies, symptoms may continue beyond 20–22 weeks.[1,2] Majority of pregnant women experience some kind of discomfort because of nausea and vomiting, and the condition is often considered to have functional overtones. The sickness in normal pregnant women may be an evolutionary protective mechanism, causing women to physically vomit and develop dislike for foods that are likely to be toxic to the embryo like caffeinated beverages and alcohol. This theory is supported by studies showing that women who had nausea and vomiting were less likely to have miscarriages and stillbirth.[3,4]

Hyperemesis gravidarum is characterized by persistent and intractable nausea and vomiting associated with ketosis and weight loss (>5% of prepregnancy weight). Hyperemesis gravidarum may, in turn, cause volume depletion, electrolytes and acid-base imbalances, nutritional deficiencies, and even death. Severe hyperemesis requiring hospital admission occurs in 0.3–2% of pregnancies.[5] Like nausea and vomiting during pregnancy, hyperemesis also typically starts before the 10th week and resolves by 20 weeks of gestation, with the symptoms at peak by 14 weeks. In about 10% of patients, symptoms may persist throughout the course of pregnancy.

Hyperemesis gravidarum is commonly believed to be of no major consequence. However, before intravenous fluids were available, it was an important cause of maternal morbidity. Even with all the medical advances, fatal complications like Wernicke's encephalopathy, central pontine myelinolysis, vasospasm of the cerebral arteries leading to stroke, rhabdomyolysis, and coagulopathy have been reported in literature.[6-9]

PATHOPHYSIOLOGY OF HYPEREMESIS GRAVIDARUM

Hyperemesis gravidarum appears to occur as a complex interaction of biological, psychological, and sociocultural factors. The physiologic basis of hyperemesis gravidarum is controversial. The hypothesis that endocrine factors are the most important has primarily developed because the peak symptoms of hyperemesis gravidarum happen during early pregnancy—the time when the placenta and the corpus luteum are producing increased levels of hormones.

HORMONAL CHANGES

Human Chorionic Gonadotropin

Human chorionic gonadotropin (hCG) is cited as the most likely cause of hyperemesis gravidarum, either directly or through its action on the thyroid-stimulating hormone (TSH) receptors.

Evidence in Favor

- The highest incidence of hyperemesis gravidarum coincides with the time when hCG levels are at the highest during pregnancy
- Higher incidence of hyperemesis gravidarum has been reported by various authors in conditions, which are known to be associated with higher hCG levels like twin pregnancies,[10] molar pregnancies,[11] pregnancies with female fetuses,[12] and in mothers bearing children with Down syndrome[13]
- Over 11 different studies have shown significantly higher levels of hCG in women with hyperemesis gravidarum, compared to age and gestational age-matched controls.[14]

Proposed Mechanisms of Hyperemesis Gravidarum by hCG

The pathway in which higher levels of hCG leads to hyperemesis gravidarum is still unclear, but the proposed mechanisms include activation of secretory process in the upper gastrointestinal (GI) tract and by the stimulation of increased thyroid hormone production by hCG,[15] as summarized in figure 7-1.

Evidence Against

- Not all conditions with high hCG levels are associated with hyperemesis gravidarum, e.g., choriocarcinoma
- Many women with high hCG levels do not have symptoms associated with nausea and vomiting in pregnancy or hyperemesis gravidarum
- Over 10% of patients continue to be symptomatic even after 20 weeks when the levels of hCG start to fall
- During treatment with parenteral hCG used for oocyte maturation in patients with infertility, there is no increase in the incidence of nausea or vomiting.

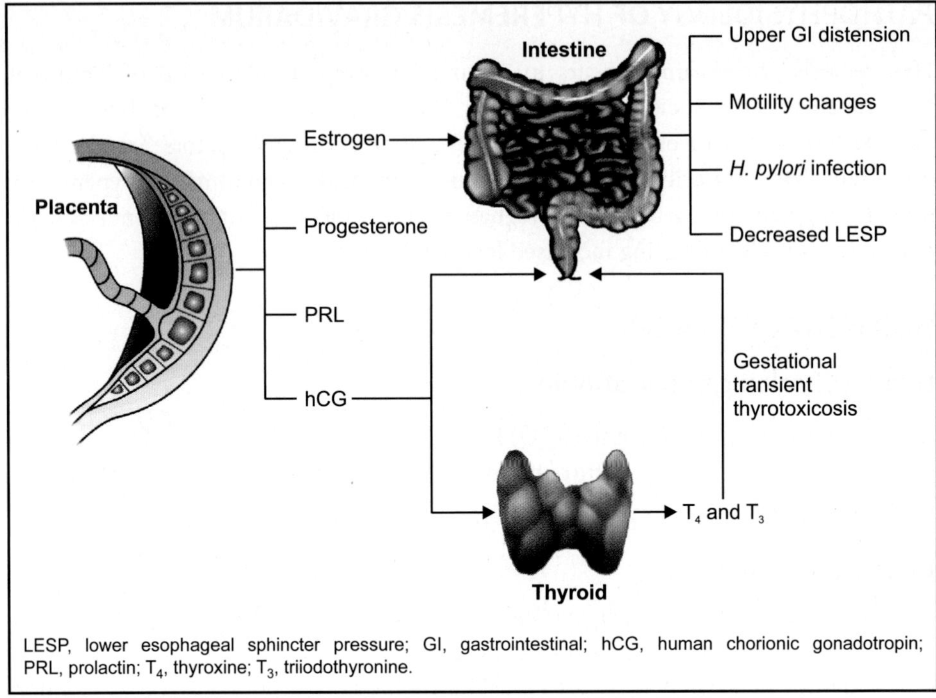

Figure 7-1 Interactions between various hormones and target organs possibly involved in the pathogenesis of hyperemesis gravidarum.

Some of these dissenting results have been explained by the fact that it may not be the absolute increase in hCG itself that is responsible for nausea and vomiting in pregnancy, but an increase in specific subtype of hCG that is more important. These isoforms are more sialylated with asialo-carbohydrates and are found towards more acidic pH when chromatographed.[16,17] These differences may be inherent to communities, either via the genes or through environmental conditioning and help in explaining why Indian and Pakistani women in the UK have more chances of developing hyperemesis gravidarum than ethnic European women.[19]

Progesterone

The production of progesterone from corpus luteum is highest during the first trimester, when the incidence of hyperemesis gravidarum is highest.

Evidence in Favor

- The evidence is less convincing with several researchers having found low progesterone levels associated with hyperemesis gravidarum and the others having found higher levels associated with hyperemesis gravidarum[14]

Evidence Against

- The inconsistent results of various studies looking at the role of progesterone in hyperemesis gravidarum is the main evidence against this theory
- Treatment of patients with hyperemesis gravidarum with progesterone did not alleviate symptoms when administered in a prospective cohort study[19]
- Other conditions with iatrogenic high progesterone levels like ovarian hyperstimulation did not result in an increase in nausea.[14]

Estrogen

Evidence in Favor

- Several conditions, which are associated with high estrogen levels in pregnancy are associated with an increase in hyperemesis gravidarum like obesity[20] and primigravida[19]
- Nausea is a common side effect of estrogen treatment amongst women using it as a contraceptive
- A delivery outcome study in women with hyperemesis gravidarum revealed higher incidence of congenital malformations: undescended testicles, hip dysplasia, and Down syndrome[21]
- Some studies have shown an increase in estrogen when compared to controls in patients with hyperemesis gravidarum[14]
- A retrospective study has shown that women with hyperemesis gravidarum and nausea and vomiting in pregnancy are more likely to suffer from nausea when given estrogen containing contraceptive pills, supporting the hypothesis that some women are more sensitive to the effects of estrogen on the intestines.[22]

Proposed Mechanisms of Hyperemesis Gravidarum by Estrogen

Estrogen has multiple effects on the GI tract. High levels of estrogen cause slower intestinal transit time and directly inhibit gastric emptying. When accompanied by its ability to retain fluids, they cause accumulation of fluids in the GI tract. Another proposed mechanism is that an estrogen-led shift in upper intestinal pH leads to manifestations of subclinical *Helicobacter pylori* infection (Figure 7-1).[23,24]

Evidence Against

- The main argument against estrogen, however, is that it does not explain the temporal profile of the disease, as to why the disease is mostly limited and worse during the first trimester, while the levels progressively rise during the course of pregnancy
- Pregnancies induced by ovarian hyperstimulation in assisted reproduction, when the circulating estrogen levels are very high, are not associated with a higher incidence of hyperemesis gravidarum.

Thyroid Hormones

Thyroid gland is physiologically stimulated during pregnancy, as described in detail in Chapter 1: Endocrine Physiology in Pregnancy. When there is an increase in free thyroid hormones above the trimester-specific upper limits transiently with some symptoms, the state is referred as gestational transient thyrotoxicosis.

Evidence in Favor

- Over two-thirds of pregnancies with hyperemesis gravidarum also have gestational transient thyrotoxicosis[25]
- Patients suffering from hyperemesis gravidarum had consistently higher levels of free thyoxine (T_4) in over 8 gestational age-matched studies when compared to controls[14]
- Free T_4 levels have also been correlated with the severity of symptoms in patients with hyperemesis gravidarum.[25]

Evidence Against

- Only 70% of patients with hyperemesis gravidarum have suppressed TSH levels[25]
- Other diseases with increased thyroid hormones like Graves' disease, are not associated with an increase in nausea and vomiting in pregnancy or hyperemesis gravidarum
- Many patients with gestational transient thyrotoxicosis have no symptoms of hyperemesis gravidarum.

Despite the inconclusive evidence, as to if gestational transient thyrotoxicosis and hyperemesis gravidarum being causal or part of the same syndrome, there is an increasing recognition that hypersensitivity to the actions of hCG on TSH receptors even with normal circulation levels can happen through 2 mechanisms:

- Hypersensitive TSH receptors on the thyroid gland to hCG were observed in a family with gestational transient thyrotoxicosis and hyperemesis gravidarum. A mutation on the extracellular domain of the TSH receptor made the receptor more susceptible to normal circulating levels of hCG[26]
- On the other hand, isoforms of hCG, especially the isoforms containing asialo-carbohydrate chains, are more potent in the stimulation of TSH receptor than native hCG and this, in turn, could explain the coincidence of hyperemesis gravidarum and gestational transient thyrotoxicosis.[17,27]

Leptin

The recent finding that leptin is expressed in the placenta and elevated leptin levels accompany several pregnancy-related disorders like preeclampsia and gestational diabetes, brought attention to the role of leptin in hyperemesis gravidarum.[14]

However, 3 studies looking prospectively at serum leptin levels and hyperemesis gravidarum did not find any statistically significant difference. But some studies revealed that this was likely to be false-negative, as most conditions involving starvation and vomiting should result in a dramatic decrease in leptin levels which was not seen in these cases.[28]

Adrenal Cortex

Steroid therapy is one of the oldest therapies for hyperemesis gravidarum and has been used since 1950s. This led to the hypothesis that adrenal cortical deficiency leads to symptoms of hyperemesis gravidarum. A single study also reported significantly lower cortisol levels in patients with hyperemesis gravidarum.[29] However, recent studies have all shown that instead of lower cortisol levels, there is an upregulation of hypothalamic-pituitary-adrenal axis with increased levels of adrenocorticotropic hormone (ACTH) and cortisol.[14] Moreover, this appears protective in nature and a meta-analysis of the randomized controlled trials using steroids did not demonstrate that steroids relieve symptoms.[30]

NONHORMONAL CHANGES

Gastrointestinal Dysfunction

Gastric dysrhythmias have been shown to be associated with morning sickness. The presence of dysrhythmias is associated with nausea, while normal myoelectrical activity is present in the absence of nausea. Mechanisms that cause gastric dysrhythmias include elevated estrogen or progesterone levels, thyroid disorders, abnormalities in vagal and sympathetic tone, and vasopressin secretion in response to intravascular volume perturbation. Many of which are present in early pregnancy.[31]

Hepatic Dysfunction

Impairment of mitochondrial fatty acid oxidation has been hypothesized to play a role in the pathogenesis of maternal liver disease associated with hyperemesis gravidarum. Fatty acid oxidation defects develop in hyperemesis gravidarum due to accumulation of fatty acids in the placenta and subsequent generation of reactive oxygen species. Also, starvation leading to peripheral lipolysis and increased load of fatty acids in maternal-fetal circulation, combined with reduced capacity of the mitochondria to oxidize fatty acids in mothers heterozygous for fatty acid oxidation defects, can cause hyperemesis gravidarum and liver injury.[32]

Lipid Alterations

Levels of triglycerides, total cholesterol, and phospholipids vary in women with hyperemesis gravidarum. This may be related to the abnormalities in hepatic function in pregnant women as compared to controls.[33]

Infection

H. pylori, found in the stomach, may aggravate nausea and vomiting in pregnancy. Studies have found conflicting evidence of the role of *H. pylori* in hyperemesis gravidarum. However, persistent nausea and vomiting beyond the second trimester may be due to an active peptic ulcer caused by *H. pylori* infection.[34,35]

Vestibular Disorders and Olfactory Hyperacuity

Many pregnant women report that the smell of cooking food, particularly meat, triggers the nausea. Hyperacuity of the olfactory system may be a contributing factor to nausea and vomiting during pregnancy. Similarities between hyperemesis gravidarum and motion sickness suggest that unmasking of subclinical vestibular disorders may account for some cases of hyperemesis gravidarum.[36,37]

Genetic

Data suggest that a genetic predisposition may play a role in the development of hyperemesis gravidarum. Women who were born after an unaffected pregnancy had a risk of 1.1%. Mothers who had pregnancies complicated by hyperemesis gravidarum also reported higher rates of hyperemesis gravidarum among their relatives, especially in their sisters.[38,39]

Immunological

Hyperemesis gravidarum is associated with overactivation of sympathetic nerves and enhanced production of tumor necrosis factor (TNF)-α.[40] Increased adenosine levels have also been noted; since adenosine is an established suppressor of excessive sympathetic nerves activation and cytokine production, the increase in plasma adenosine in hyperemesis gravidarum may be modulatory.[41] Trophoblast-derived cytokines have been reported to induce secretion of hCG.

Immunoglobulins, C3 and C4, and lymphocyte counts are significantly higher in women with hyperemesis gravidarum. Type 1 T helper (Th1)/Type 2 T helper (Th2) cells balance is decreased in women with hyperemesis gravidarum, which results in increased humoral immunity. Increased fetal DNA has been found in the plasma of women with hyperemesis gravidarum, and the increased DNA is speculated to be derived from trophoblasts that have been destroyed by the hyperactive maternal immune system. Thus, hyperemesis gravidarum may be mediated by immunologic aberrations in pregnancy.[42-45]

Psychological Issues

Physiological changes associated with pregnancy interact with a woman's psychological state and cultural values. Psychological responses may interact with and exacerbate the physiology of nausea and vomiting during pregnancy. Nonetheless, hyperemesis gravidarum is typically the cause of, as opposed to the result of, psychological stress. In very unusual instances, cases of hyperemesis gravidarum could represent psychiatric illness, including conversion or somatization disorder or major depression.[46-48]

CLINICAL SYMPTOMS

Defining symptoms of hyperemesis gravidarum are nausea and vomiting. Other common symptoms include ptyalism (excessive salivation), fatigue, weakness, and dizziness. Patients may experience sleep disturbance, hyperolfaction, dysgeusia (distorted sense of taste), decreased gustatory discernment, depression, anxiety, irritability, and mood changes.

RISK FACTORS

- Previous pregnancies with hyperemesis gravidarum
- Greater body weight
- Multiple gestations
- Trophoblastic disease
- Nulliparity.

INVESTIGATIONS

- Urinalysis for ketones and specific gravity: Ketones in urine, a sign of starvation, may be harmful to fetal development. High specific gravity occurs with volume depletion
- Serum electrolytes and ketones: Assess electrolyte status to evaluate for low potassium or sodium, identify hyperchloremic metabolic alkalosis or acidosis, and evaluate renal function for volume status
- Liver enzymes and bilirubin: Elevated transaminase levels may occur in as many as 50% of patients with hyperemesis gravidarum. Mild transaminitis often resolves once the nausea has resolved. Significantly elevated liver enzymes, however, may be a sign of another underlying liver condition, such as hepatitis (viral, ischemic, autoimmune), or some other etiology of liver injury[49]
- Amylase/lipase: Amylase level is elevated in approximately 10% of patients with hyperemesis gravidarum. Lipase, when combined with amylase, can increase the specificity in diagnosing pancreatitis as an etiology
- TSH, free T_4: Hyperemesis gravidarum is often associated with a transient hyperthyroidism and suppressed TSH levels in 50–60% of cases. However, an elevated

free T_4 may suggest that overt hyperthyroidism is present, thus, necessitating a further workup and treatment[50]

- Urine culture: This may be indicated because urinary tract infection is common in pregnancy and can be associated with nausea and vomiting
- Calcium level: Consider measuring Ca^{2+} levels. Some rare cases have been reported of hypercalcemia being associated with hyperemesis gravidarum, resulting from hyperparathyroidism
- Hematocrit: This may be elevated because of volume contraction.

MANAGEMENT

Initial management should be conservative and may include reassurance, dietary recommendations, and support. Alternative therapies may include acupressure and hypnosis. Psychological counseling may be considered.[50] Outpatient or home intravenous hydration should be considered. If medications and outpatient hydration fail or if severe electrolyte disturbances persist, inpatient admission for intravenous hydration may be necessary.

PHARMACOLOGIC THERAPY

- Treatment may be initiated using vitamin B6, 10–25 mg, 3–4 times daily; doxylamine, 12.5 mg, 3–4 times daily can be used in addition
- The herb, ginger capsules 250 mg 4 times daily, can be added at this point if the patient is still vomiting, since it has been shown to be effective in randomized trials[52]
- Metoclopramide, 5–10 mg taken orally thrice a day may be used next
- Promethazine, 12.5 mg orally or rectally 4 times a day, or dimenhydrinate 50–100 mg orally every 4–6 hours, may be added as well
- Ondansetron 4–8 mg orally or intravenously thrice a day can be used for further refractory cases
- Methylprednisolone, 16 mg orally or intravenously thrice a day for 3 days, with a taper to lowest effective dose, can be used if persistent vomiting occurs despite the above therapy. This should be one of the last resorts, since steroids seem to increase the risk for oral clefts in first 10 weeks of gestation[53]
- In case of severe or symptomatic hypokalemia, potassium should be replaced parenterally
- If persistent dehydration, electrolyte loss, and/or weight loss occur despite above therapy, nutrition supplementation by either parenteral or enteral route is indicated.

In some refractory severe cases of hyperemesis gravidarum, if maternal survival is threatened, or if hyperemesis gravidarum is causing severe physical and psychological burden termination of pregnancy should be considered.[54]

PREVENTIVE MEASURES

Early patient education, knowledge about pregnancy, stress, doubts regarding the pregnancy, and good communication with the doctor and spouse is necessary. Early interventions include reassurance and dietary counseling, advising the patient to eat small meals, to avoid high-fat or spicy foods, to follow hunger cues, and to increase the intake of dry carbohydrates and carbonated beverages.

CONCLUSION

Nausea and vomiting are one of the most common symptoms of early pregnancy. Although, hyperemesis gravidarum presents itself as a serious condition, availability of better management and fluid replacement nowadays, maternal morbidity rate due to hyperemesis has decreased to a major extent. An interplay of various physiological, psychological, and sociocultural factors lead to hyperemesis gravidarum in a small proportion of pregnant women. Preventive measures need to be taken early, as soon as the pregnancy is confirmed. After diagnosis, prompt medical assistance and appropriate management need to be provided in order to ensure safe progression of pregnancy.

REFERENCES

1. Lacroix R, Eason E, Melzack R. Nausea and vomiting during pregnancy: A prospective study of its frequency, intensity, and patterns of change. *Am J Obstet Gynecol.* 2000;182: 931-7.
2. Bailit JL. Hyperemesis gravidarum: Epidemiologic findings from a large cohort. *Am J Obstet Gynecol.* 2005;193:811-4.
3. Sherman PW, Flaxman SM. Nausea and vomiting of pregnancy in an evolutionary perspective. *Am J Obstet Gynecol.* 2002;186:190-7.
4. Creasy RK, Resnik R. Gastrointestinal disease in pregnancy. In: Creasy RK, Resnik R, eds. Maternal-Fetal Medicine, Principles and Practice. 5th ed. Philadelphia, Pa: WB Saunders; 2004. p. 1109-22.
5. Goodwin TM. Hyperemesis gravidarum. *Obstet Gynecol Clin North Am.* 2008;35:401-17.
6. Peeters A, Van de Wyngaert F, Van Lierde M, Sindic CJ, Laterre EC. Wernicke's encephalopathy and central pontine myelinolysis induced by hyperemesis gravidarum. *Acta Neurol Belg.* 1993;93:276-82.
7. Kanayama N, Khatun S, Belayet HM, Yamashita M, Yonezawa M, Kobayashi T, et al. Vasospasms of cerebral arteries in hyperemesis gravidarum. *Gynecol Obstet Invest.* 1998;46:139-41.
8. Robinson JN, Banerjee R, Thiet MP. Coagulopathy secondary to vitamin K deficiency in hyperemesis gravidarum. *Obstet Gynecol.* 1998;92:673-5.
9. Togay-Isikay C, Yigit A, Mutluer N. Wernicke's encephalopathy due to hyperemesis gravidarum: an under-recognised condition. *Aust N Z J Obstet Gynaecol.* 2001;41:453-6.

10. Steier JA, Bergsjo PB, Thorsen T, Myking OL. Human chorionic gonadotropin in maternal serum in relation to fetal gender and utero-placental blood flow. *Acta Obstet Gynecol Scand.* 2004;83:170-4.
11. Basso O, Olsen J. Sex ratio and twinning in women with hyperemesis or pre-eclampsia. *Epidemiology.* 2001;12:747-9.
12. Danzer H, Braustein GD, Rasor J, Forsythe A, Wade ME. Maternal serum human chorionic gonadotropin concentrations and fetal sex prediction. *Fertil Steril.* 1980;34:336-40.
13. Askling J, Erlandsson G, Kaijser M, Akre O, Ekbom A. Sickness in pregnancy and sex of child. *Lancet.* 1999;354:2053.
14. Verberg MF, Gillott DJ, Al-Fardan N, Grudzinskas JG. Hyperemesis gravidarum, a literature review. *Hum Reprod Update.* 2005;11:527-39.
15. Hershman JM. Physiological and pathological aspects of the effect of human chorionic gonadotropin on the thyroid. *Best Pract Res Clin Endocrinol Metab.* 2004;18:249-65.
16. Jordan V, Grebe SK, Cooke RR, Ford HC, Larsen PD, Stone PR, et al. Acidic isoforms of chorionic gonadotrophin in European and Samoan women are associated with hyperemesis gravidarum and may be thyrotrophic. *Clin Endocrinol (Oxf).* 1999;50:619-27.
17. Tsuruta E, Tada H, Tamaki H, Kashiwai T, Asahi K, Takeoka K, et al. Pathogenic role of asialo human chorionic gonadotropin in gestational thyrotoxicosis. *J Clin Endocrinol Metab.* 1995;80:350-5.
18. Price A, Daviers R, Heller ST, Milford-Ward A, Weetman AP. Asian women are at increased risk of gestational thyrotoxicosis. *J Clin Endocrinol Metab.* 1996;81:1160-3.
19. Fairweather DV. Nausea and vomiting in pregnancy. *Am J Obstet Gynecol.* 1968;102:135-75.
20. Depue RH, Bernstein L, Ross RK, Judd HL, Henderson BE. Hyperemesis gravidarum in relation to estradiol levels, pregnancy outcome, and other maternal factors: a sero-epidemiologic study. *Am J Obstet Gynecol.* 1987;156:1137-41.
21. Kallen B. Hyperemesis during pregnancy and delivery outcome: a registry study. *Eur J Obstet Gynecol Reprod Biol.* 1987;26:291-302.
22. Jarnfelt-Samsioe A, Samsioe G, Velinder GM. Nausea and vomiting in pregnancy – a contribution to its epidemiology. *Gynecol Obstet Invest.* 1983;16:221-9.
23. Walsh JW, Hasler WL, Nugent CE, Owyang C. Progesterone and estrogen are potential mediators of gastric slow-wave dysrhythmias in nausea of pregnancy. *Am J Physiol.* 1996; 270:G506-14.
24. Kocak I, Akcan Y, Ustun C, Demirel C, Cengiz L, Yanik FF. Helicobacter pylori seropositivity in patients with hyperemesis gravidarum. *Int J Gynaecol Obstet.* 1999;66:251-4.
25. Goodwin TM, Montoro M, Mestman JH. Transient hyperthyroidism and hyperemesis gravidarum: clinical aspects. *Am J Obstet Gynecol.* 1992;167:648-52.
26. Rodien P, Jordan N, Lefevre A, Royer J, Vasseur C, Savagner F, et al. Abnormal stimulation of the thyrotrophin receptor during gestation. *Hum Reprod Update.* 2004;10:95-105.
27. Yamazaki K, Sato K, Shizume K, Kanaji Y, Ito Y, Obara T, et al. Potent thyrotropic activity of human chorionic gonadotropin variants in terms of 125I incorporation and denovo synthesized thyroid hormone release in human thyroid follicles. *J Clin Endocrinol Metab.* 1995;80:473-9.
28. Boden G, Chen X, Mozzoli M, Ryani I. Effect of fasting on serum leptin in normal human subjects. *J Clin Endocrinol Metab.* 1996;81:3419-23.

29. Jarnfelt-Samsioe A, Bremme K, Eneroth P. Steroid hormones in emetic and non-emetic pregnancy. *Eur J Obstet Gynecol Reprod Biol.* 1986;21:87-99.
30. Jewell D, Young G. Interventions for nausea and vomiting in early pregnancy. *Cochrane Database Syst Rev.* 2003;(4):CD000145.
31. Koch KL. Gastrointestinal factors in nausea and vomiting of pregnancy. *Am J Obstet Gynecol.* 2002;186:S198-203.
32. Jarnfelt-Samsioe A, Eriksson B, Waldenstrom J, Samisoe G. Serum bile acids, gamma-glutamyltransferase and routine liver function tests in emetic and non-emetic pregnancies. *Gynecol Obstet Invest.* 1986;21:169-76.
33. Ustun Y, Engin-Ustun Y, Dokmeci F, Soylemez F. Serum concentrations of lipids and apolipoproteins in normal and hyperemetic pregnancies. *J Matern Fetal Neonatal Med.* 2004;15:287-90.
34. Kocak I, Akcan Y, Ustun C, Demiral C, Cengiz L, Yanik FF. Helicobacter pylori seropositivity in patients with hyperemesis gravidarum. *Obstet Gynecol Sur.* 2000;55:198-9.
35. Lee RH, Pan VL, Wing DA. The prevalence of Helicobacter pylori in the Hispanic population affected by hyperemesis gravidarum. *Am J Obstet Gynecol.* 2005;193:1024-7.
36. Black FO. Maternal susceptibility to nausea and vomiting of pregnancy: is the vestibular system involved? *Am J Obstet Gynecol.* 2002;186:204-9.
37. Heinrichs L. Linking olfaction with nausea and vomiting of pregnancy, recurrent abortion, hyperemesis gravidarum, and migraine headache. *Am J Obstet Gynecol.* 2002;186:215-9.
38. Vikanes A, Skjaerven R, Grjibovski AM, Gunnes N, Vangen S, Magnus P. Recurrence of hyperemesis gravidarum across generations: population based cohort study. *BMJ.* 2010; 340:c2050.
39. Zhang Y, Cantor RM, MacGibbon K, Romero R, Goodwin TM, Mullin PM, et al. Familial aggregation of hyperemesis gravidarum. *Am J Obstet Gynecol.* 2011;204:230.
40. Kaplan PB, Gucer F, Sayin NC, Yuksel M, Yuce MA, Yardin T. Maternal serum cytokine levels in women with hyperemesis gravidarum in the first trimester of pregnancy. *Fertil Steril.* 2003;79:498-502.
41. Kiyokawa Y, Yoneyama Y. Relationship between adenosine and T-helper 1/T-helper 2 balance in hyperemesis gravidarum. *Clin Chim Acta.* 2006;370:137-42.
42. Sekizawa A, Sugito Y, Iwasaki M, Watanabe A, Jimbo M, Hoshi S, et al. Cell-free fetal DNA is increased in plasma of women with hyperemesis gravidarum. *Clin Chem.* 2001;47:2164-5.
43. Sugito Y, Sekizawa A, Farina A, Yukimoto Y, Saito H, Iwasaki M, et al. Relationship between severity of hyperemesis gravidarum and fetal DNA concentration in maternal plasma. *Clin Chem.* 2003;49:1667-9.
44. Yoneyama Y, Suzuki S, Sawa R, Araki T. Plasma adenosine concentrations increase in women with hyperemesis gravidarum. *Clin Chim Acta.* 2005;352:75-9.
45. Yoneyama Y, Suzuki S, Sawa R, Yoneyama K, Doi D, Otusbo Y, et al. The T-helper 1/ T-helper 2 balance in peripheral blood of women with hyperemesis gravidarum. *Am J Obstet Gynecol.* 2002;187:1631-5.
46. Simpson SW, Goodwin TM, Robins SB, Rizzo AA, Howes RA, Buckwalter DK, et al. Psychological factors and hyperemesis gravidarum. *J Womens Health Gend Based Med.* 2001;10:471-7.

47. Buckwalter JG, Simpson SW. Psychological factors in the etiology and treatment of severe nausea and vomiting in pregnancy. *Am J Obstet Gynecol.* 2002;186:210-4.
48. Morrow GR, Roscoe JA, Hickok JT, Andrews PR, Matterson S. Nausea and emesis: evidence for a bio behavioral perspective. *Support Care Cancer.* 2002;10:96-105.
49. Hay JE. Liver disease in pregnancy. *Hepatology.* 2008;47:1067-76.
50. Tan JY, Loh KC, Yeo GS, Chee YC. Transient hyperthyroidism of hyperemesis gravidarum. *BJOG.* 2002;109:683-8.
51. Simon EP, Schwartz J. Medical hypnosis for hyperemesis gravidarum. *Birth.* 1999;26: 248-54.
52. Borrelli F, Capasso R, Aviello G, Pittler MH, Izzo AA. Effectiveness and safety of ginger in the treatment of pregnancy-induced nausea and vomiting. *Obstet Gynecol.* 2005;105: 849-56.
53. Safari HR, Alsulyman OM, Gherman RB, Goodwin TM. Experience with oral methyl-prednisolone in the treatment of refractory hyperemesis gravidarum. *Am J Obstet Gynecol.* 1998;178:1054-8.
54. Poursharif B, Korst LM, Macgibbon KW, Feizo MS, Romero R, Goodwin TM. Elective pregnancy termination in a large cohort of women with hyperemesis gravidarum. *Contraception.* 2007;76:451-5.

8

Hypertension and Pregnancy

Rajesh Rajput

INTRODUCTION

Hypertension is the most common disorder complicating 5–10% of pregnancies and remains a leading cause of maternal and fetal morbidity and mortality.[1] The various maternal complications include increased chances of abruptio placentae, cerebrovascular accidents, disseminated intravascular complications, and various end organ failure while fetal complications include intrauterine growth retardation (IUGR), prematurity, and intrauterine deaths.[1-3]

CHRONIC AND GESTATIONAL HYPERTENSION

Chronic hypertension is defined as blood pressure exceeding 140/90 mmHg before pregnancy or before 20 weeks of gestation, if identified for the first time during the pregnancy.[2] In contrast, gestational hypertension is defined as new onset of elevated blood pressure after 20 weeks of gestation and followed by normalization of the blood pressure postpartum.[3] With increasing prevalence of obesity, both chronic hypertension and gestational hypertension are now increasingly recognized. Chronic hypertension is essential (90–95%) or primary in majority of cases while in 5–10% of cases, it is secondary to renal parenchymal or vascular diseases and various endocrine disorders like Cushing's syndrome, pheochromocytoma, hyperthyroidism, hypothyroidism, and hyperparathyroidism.[3,4] As recommended by the National High Blood Pressure Education Program (NHBPEP) Working Group[3] on high blood pressure in pregnancy, hypertensive disorders during pregnancy are classified into 4 categories (Table 8-1).

In women with preexisting hypertension, preeclampsia should be defined as resistant hypertension, new or worsening proteinuria, or one or more of the other adverse conditions. In women with gestational hypertension, preeclampsia should be defined as new-onset proteinuria or one or more of the other adverse conditions, such

TABLE 8-1

Classification of Hypertensive Disorders During Pregnancy—National High Blood Pressure Education Program Working Group on High Blood Pressure in Pregnancy	
Primary diagnosis	*Definition of preeclampsia*
Preexisting hypertension	
• Without comorbid conditions • With comorbid conditions (like diabetes, renal disease, or taking antihypertensive therapy outside pregnancy for any reason) • Preeclampsia-eclampsia (after 20 weeks of gestation).	Resistant hypertension, or new worsening proteinuria, or one/more adverse condition(s) as mentioned in text
Gestational hypertension	
• Without comorbid conditions • With comorbid conditions (like diabetes, renal disease, or taking antihypertensive therapy outside pregnancy for any reason) • Preeclampsia-eclampsia (after 20 weeks of gestation).	New worsening proteinuria, or one/more adverse condition(s) as mentioned in text

Source: Report of the National High Blood Pressure Education Program Working Group on High Blood Pressure in Pregnancy. *Am J Obstet Gynecol*. 2000;183:S1-S22.

as maternal symptoms like persistent or new/unusual headache, visual disturbances, persistent abdominal or right upper quadrant pain, severe nausea or vomiting, chest pain or dyspnea, maternal signs of end-organ dysfunction like eclampsia, severe hypertension, pulmonary edema, or suspected placental abruption, abnormal maternal laboratory test results [elevated serum creatinine (according to local laboratory criteria); elevated aspartate transaminase (AST), alanine transaminase (ALT), or lactate dehydrogenase (LDH) with symptoms; platelet count $<100 \times 10^9$/L; serum albumin <20 g/L)], or fetal morbidity like oligohydramnios, IUGR, absent or reversed end-diastolic flow in the umbilical artery by Doppler velocimetry, or intrauterine fetal death.

In addition, once diagnosed, hypertension should be classified as mild, moderate, and severe hypertension (Table 8-2).

TABLE 8-2

Subclassification of Hypertension During Pregnancy		
	Systolic blood pressure (mmHg)	*Diastolic blood pressure (mmHg)*
Mild hypertension	140–149	90–99
Moderate hypertension	150–159	100–109
Severe hypertension	≥160	≥110

Isolated systolic blood pressure was previously excluded from the definition of hypertension in pregnancy for several reasons. However, even an intermittently elevated systolic blood pressure is a risk marker for later development of gestational hypertension, therefore, systolic blood pressure above 140 mmHg should trigger a closer follow-up and appropriate investigations. Isolated office hypertension i.e., white coat hypertension should be defined as office diastolic blood pressure of 90 mmHg, but home blood pressure below 135/85 mmHg. Ideally, normal home blood pressure values should be confirmed by 24-hour ambulatory blood pressure monitoring.

BLOOD PRESSURE MEASURING DURING PREGNANCY

The procedure to measure blood pressure in pregnant women is not different from that in nonpregnant women.[4,5] The recommendations for measuring blood pressure are summarized in table 8-3.

PATHOPHYSIOLOGY

The exact pathophysiology of gestational hypertension is unknown, but in the absence of features of preeclampsia, maternal and fetal outcomes are usually normal. Gestational hypertension may, however, be a harbinger of chronic hypertension later in life.

TABLE 8-3

Recommendations for Measuring Blood Pressure During Pregnancy
• Blood pressure should be measured with the woman in the sitting position with arm at the level of the heart
• An appropriately sized cuff (i.e., length of 1.5 times the circumference of the arm) should be used
• Korotkoff phase V should be used to designate diastolic blood pressure
• If blood pressure is consistently higher in one arm, the arm with the higher values should be used for all blood pressure measurements
• Blood pressure can be measured using a mercury sphygmomanometer, calibrated aneroid device, or an automated blood pressure device that has been validated for use in preeclampsia
• Automated blood pressure machines may underestimate blood pressure in women with preeclampsia and comparison of readings using mercury sphygmomanometer or an aneroid device is recommended
• Ambulatory blood pressure monitoring (by 24-hour home measurement) may be useful to detect isolated office (white coat) hypertension
• Patients should be instructed on proper blood pressure measurement technique if they are to perform home blood pressure monitoring.

Source: Hemmelgarn BR, McAlister FA, Grover S, Myers MG, McKay DW, Bolli P, et al. The 2006 Canadian Hypertension Education Program recommendations for the management of hypertension: Part I—Blood pressure measurement, diagnosis and assessment of risk. *Can J Cardiol.* 2006;22:573-81.

TABLE 8-4

Risk Factors Associated with Preeclampsia		
Maternal personal risk factors	*Maternal medical risk factors*	*Placental/fetal risk factors*
• First pregnancy • Age younger than 18 years or older than 35 years • History of preeclampsia • Family history of preeclampsia in a first-degree relative • Black race • Obesity (BMI ≥30) • Interpregnancy interval less than 2 years or longer than 10 years.	• Chronic hypertension • Preexisting type 1 or type 2 diabetes, especially with microvascular disease • Renal disease • Systemic lupus erythematosus • Obesity • Thrombophilia • History of migraine.	• Multiple gestations • Hydrops fetalis • Gestational trophoblastic disease • Triploidy.

BMI, body mass index.

In all women with pregnancy and hypertension, the presence or absence of preeclampsia must be ascertained; given its clear association with more adverse maternal and perinatal outcomes. Women with preexisting hypertension have a 10–20% risk of developing preeclampsia, while women with gestational hypertension with onset before 34 weeks are more likely to develop preeclampsia as opposed to those having its onset after 34 weeks. Preeclampsia is primarily a disorder of placental dysfunction leading to a syndrome of endothelial dysfunction with associated vasospasm. The widespread endothelial dysfunction may manifest as a maternal syndrome, fetal syndrome, or both. The various risk factors associated with development of preeclampsia are summarized in table 8-4.[6-8]

INVESTIGATIONS

For women with preexisting hypertension, serum creatinine, plasma glucose, serum potassium, urinalysis for spot/24-hour protein excretion, AST, ALT, and serum LDH should be performed in early pregnancy, if not done previously. Additional laboratory work-up should be advised depending on the presence or absence of various comorbid conditions. Women with suspected preeclampsia should undergo additional maternal and fetal testing, which include peripheral blood film examination for evidence of microangiopathy with fragmented red blood cells (RBCs), activated partial thromboplastin time (aPTT), and international normalized ratio (INR) for underlying disseminated intravascular coagulation (DIC), and fetal ultrasonographic assessment for assessment of intrauterine fetal growth and umbilical artery Doppler examination.[3,4]

TREATMENT

The aim of treatment of hypertension in pregnancy is not to cure preeclampsia but to prevent cerebral hemorrhage and eclampsia and, perhaps, delay progression of proteinuria. Uncontrolled hypertension is a frequent trigger for delivery and control of hypertension may allow prolongation of pregnancy. There is a general consensus that severe hypertension should be treated in pregnancy to decrease maternal morbidity and mortality. Blood pressure should be lowered to less than 160 mmHg systolic and less than 110 mmHg diastolic. Initial antihypertensive therapy should be started with labetalol, nifedipine capsules or tablets, or hydralazine. Magnesium sulfate is not recommended as an antihypertensive agent. Continuous fetal heart rate monitoring is advised until blood pressure is stable. Management of a woman with mild-to-moderate hypertension, i.e., blood pressure of 140–159/90–109 mmHg is much debated. Any antihypertensive therapy, as compared to placebo or no therapy, decreases the risk of transient, severe hypertension [relative risk (RR) 0.50, 95% confidence interval (CI) 0.41–0.61, 19 trials, 2409 women; number needed to treat (NNT): 9–17], without a clear difference in other maternal or perinatal outcomes, such as stroke, perinatal death, or preterm delivery. The results of a small pilot randomized control trial and a meta-analysis of randomized trials indicate that antihypertensive therapy may even be harmful, as a significant relationship between the antihypertensive-induced fall in mean arterial pressure and the risk of small for gestational age (SGA) infants or lower birth weight has been observed. However, majority of these trials are criticized because of flaws in study design, small number of patients recruited, and starting the drug too late in pregnancy. Since there is no reliable data on long-term developmental outcomes, a large definitive trial to settle this issue is needed in future.

For women without comorbid conditions, antihypertensive drug therapy should be used to maintain systolic blood pressure at 130–155 mmHg and diastolic blood pressure at 80–105 mmHg. For women with comorbid conditions, antihypertensive drug therapy should be used to maintain systolic blood pressure at 130–139 mmHg and diastolic blood pressure at 80–89 mmHg. Medicinal therapy can be initiated with one of variety of antihypertensive agents like methyldopa, labetalol, β-blockers like acebutolol, metoprolol, pindolol, and propranolol, and calcium-channel blockers like nifedipine. Angiotensin converting enzyme inhibitors (ACEIs) and angiotensin II receptor blockers (ARBs) should not be used and their use in the third trimester has been associated with fetal death and neonatal renal failure. Sufficient data regarding safety of various newer antihypertensive drugs for treatment of hypertension during pregnancy is lacking as childbearing potential without reliable contraception is an exclusion criteria in majority of clinical trials testing these drugs.[9] The dosage and time of onset of commonly used antihypertensive drugs during pregnancy is described in table 8-5. The concern that a

TABLE 8-5

Doses of Commonly Used Agents for Treatment of Hypertension in Pregnancy		
Agent	*Dosage*	*Other comment*
Labetalol	Start with 20 mg IV; repeat 20–50 mg IV over 2 minutes or 1–2 mg/min; max. 300 mg (onset of action 5 minutes; repeat after 15–30 minutes), then switch to 100–400 mg orally BD or TDS (max. 1200 mg/day)	Side effects: nausea, headache, bradycardia, bronchospasm, scalp tingling (self-limiting, resolves in 24–48 hours) Avoid in women with asthma or heart failure Neonatologist should be informed as parenteral labetalol may cause neonatal bradycardia
Nifedipine	5–10 mg capsule (onset of action 10–20 minutes; repeat after 30 minutes) or 10–20 mg tablet (onset of action 30–45 minutes; repeat after 45 minutes)	Side effects: headache associated with flushing, tachycardia, peripheral edema, constipation
Hydralazine	Start with 5–10 mg IV; repeat IV every 30 minutes or 0.5–10 mg/hour IV to a max. of 20 mg IV (or 30 mg IM; onset of action 20 minutes)	Side effects: flushing, headache, lupus like reaction. May increase the risk of maternal hypotension
Methyldopa	250–500 mg orally TDS or QID (max. 2 g/day; onset of action over 24 hours)	There is no evidence to support a loading dose of methyldopa Side effects: dry mouth, sedation, depression, blurring of vision
Prazosin	0.5–5 mg TDS	First dose effect, orthostatic hypertension
Clonidine	75–300 μg TDS	Withdrawal effect with clonidine

IV, intravenous; IM, intramuscular; BD, twice a day; TDS, thrice a day; QID, four times a day.

precipitous fall in blood pressure after use of intravenous antihypertensive treatment, particularly hydralazine, may impair placental perfusion resulting in fetal distress can be prevented by coadministration of a small bolus of fluid, e.g., normal saline 250 mL at the time of administration of antihypertensive therapy.[10] Persistent or refractory severe hypertension may require repeated doses of these agents. Infusion of sodium nitroprusside or glyceryl trinitrate are also effective but are recommended rarely when other treatments have failed and delivery is imminent. Since sodium nitroprusside may cause fetal cyanide and thiocyanate toxicity and transient fetal bradycardia, it should be used for a short duration with intraarterial blood pressure monitoring in

TABLE 8-6

Indications of Delivery in Women with Preeclampsia and Gestational Hypertension	
Maternal indications	
• Gestational age ≥37 weeks • Inability to control hypertension • Deteriorating platelet functions • Deteriorating liver functions • Deteriorating renal functions	• Abruptio placenta • Acute pulmonary edema • Development of eclampsia • Persistent epigastric pain, nausea, and vomiting with deteriorating liver functions.
Fetal indications	
• Severe fetal IUGR	• Non reassuring fetal status.

IUGR, intrauterine growth retardation.

a high dependency care environment to effect safe operative delivery. All the drugs classes described in table 8-5 along with ACEIs and ARBs are considered safe during breastfeeding.[11]

The decision to terminate pregnancy is based on clear "endpoints" for delivery and should be defined for each patient.[12] The timing of delivery is based upon a number of factors, maternal and/or fetal rather than a single absolute indication for delivery and are summarized in table 8-6.

For pregnant women with any severity of hypertension, vaginal delivery should be considered unless a cesarean section is required for the usual obstetric indications. If vaginal delivery is planned and the cervix is unfavorable, cervical ripening should be used to increase the chances of a successful vaginal delivery. Antihypertensive treatment should be continued throughout labor and delivery to maintain systolic blood pressure at below 160 mmHg and diastolic blood pressure at below 110 mmHg. The third stage of labor should be actively managed with oxytocin 5 units intravenously or 10 units intramuscularly, particularly in the presence of thrombocytopenia or coagulopathy. For labor and delivery, epidural analgesia is a useful adjunct to antihypertensive therapy for blood pressure control and improving renal and uteroplacental blood flow. In presence of contraindications like severe thrombocytopenia, coagulopathy, and sepsis, patient-controlled intravenous analgesia with fentanyl or remifentanil is preferred. Other drugs that are best avoided in severe preeclampsia include ergometrine (should not be given in any form), ketamine (hypertension), nonsteroidal anti-inflammatory drugs (NSAIDs), and cyclooxygenase (COX-2) specific inhibitors (impaired renal function and hypertension).[13] The treatment scheme based on National Institute for Health and Clinical Excellence (NICE) guidelines[14] for hypertension during pregnancy is summarized in table 8-7.

TABLE 8-7

Treatment Scheme Based on NICE Guidelines for Hypertension During Pregnancy			
Action	*Mild hypertension (140/90–149/99 mmHg)*	*Moderate hypertension (150/100–159/109 mmHg)*	*Severe hypertension (160/110 mmHg or higher)*
Admit to hospital	No	No	Yes, until blood pressure is 159/109 mmHg or lower
Treatment	No	With oral labetalol, α-methyldopa, nifedipine as first-line treatment to keep diastolic blood pressure between 80–100 mmHg and systolic blood pressure less than 150 mmHg	Initially use IV drugs, later on switch to oral drugs as for moderate hypertension
Measure blood pressure	Not more than once a week	At least twice a week	At least 4 times a day
Test for proteinuria	At each visit using automated reagent-strip reading device or urinary protein:creatinine ratio	At each visit using automated reagent-strip reading device or urinary protein:creatinine ratio	Daily using automated reagent-strip reading device or urinary protein:creatinine ratio
Blood tests	Only those for routine antenatal care	Kidney function electrolytes, full blood count, transaminases, bilirubin. Do not carry out further blood tests if no proteinuria at subsequent visits	Test at presentation and then monitor weekly: kidney function, electrolytes, full blood count, transaminases, bilirubin

NICE, National Institute for Health and Clinical Excellence; IV, intravenous.

Source: National Collaborating Centre for Women's and Children's Health. Hypertension in pregnancy. The management of hypertensive disorders during pregnancy. London (UK): National Institute for Health and Clinical Excellence (NICE); 2010. p.46. (Clinical guideline; no. 107).

CONCLUSION

Hypertension has emerged as one of the most prevalent complications during pregnancy. It becomes mandatory to screen pregnant women with hypertension for preeclampsia given its adverse maternal and fetal outcomes. Proper investigations should be performed to determine the extent of severity. Appropriate management is needed, especially in women with preeclampsia in order to avoid/deal with complications and for safe progression of pregnancy ensuring safety of both mother and the baby.

REFERENCES

1. Magee LA, Helewa M, Moutquin JM, von Dadelszen P; Hypertension Guideline Committee; Strategic Training Initiative in Research in the Reproductive Health Sciences (STIRRHS) Scholars. Diagnosis, evaluation, and management of the hypertensive disorders of pregnancy. *J Obstet Gynaecol Can.* 2008;30:S1-48.
2. American College of Obstetricians and Gynecologists. ACOG Practice bulletin no. 125: chronic hypertension in pregnancy. *Obstet Gynecol.* 2012;119:396.
3. Report of the National High Blood Pressure Education Program Working Group on High Blood Pressure in Pregnancy. *Am J Obstet Gynecol.* 2000;183:S1-S22.
4. Hemmelgarn BR, McAlister FA, Grover S, Myers MG, McKay DW, Bolli P, et al. The 2006 Canadian Hypertension Education Program recommendations for the management of hypertension: Part I—Blood pressure measurement, diagnosis and assessment of risk. *Can J Cardiol.* 2006;22:573-81.
5. Zuspan FP, Rayburn WF. Blood pressure self-monitoring during pregnancy: Practical considerations. *Am J Obstet Gynecol.* 1991;164:2-6.
6. Sibai BM, Lindheimer M, Hauth J, Caritis S, VanDorsten P, Klebanoff M, et al. Risk factors for preeclampsia, abruptio placentae, and adverse neonatal outcomes among women with chronic hypertension. National Institute of Child Health and Human Development Network of Maternal-Fetal Medicine Units. *N Engl J Med.* 1998;339:667-71.
7. Duckitt K, Harrington D. Risk factors for pre-eclampsia at antenatal booking: systematic review of controlled studies. *BMJ.* 2005;330:565.
8. Brown MA, Mackenzie C, Dunsmuir W, Roberts L, Ikin K, Matthews J, et al. Can we predict recurrence of pre-eclampsia or gestational hypertension? *BJOG.* 2007;114:984-93.
9. Abalos E, Duley L, Steyn DW, Henderson-Smart DJ. Antihypertensive drug therapy for mild to moderate hypertension during pregnancy. *Cochrane Database Syst Rev.* 2007;(1):CD002252.
10. Magee LA, von Dadelszen P, Chan S, Gafni A, Gruslin A, Helewa M, et al. The control of hypertension in pregnancy study pilot trial. *BJOG.* 2007;114:770.
11. Beardmore KS, Morris JM, Gallery ED. Excretion of antihypertensive medication into human breast milk: a systematic review. *Hypertens Pregnancy.* 2002;21:85-95.
12. Hall DR, Odendaal HJ, Steyn DW. Expectant management of severe pre-eclampsia in the mid-trimester. *Eur J Obstet Gynecol Reprod Biol.* 2001;96:168-72.
13. Dyer RA, Piercy JL, Reed AR. The role of the anesthetist in the management of the pre-eclamptic patient. *Curr Opin Anaesthesiol.* 2007;20:168-74.
14. National Collaborating Centre for Women's and Children's Health. Hypertension in pregnancy. The management of hypertensive disorders during pregnancy. London (UK): National Institute for Health and Clinical Excellence (NICE); 2010. p.46. (Clinical guideline; no. 107).

9

Vitamin D and Pregnancy

Sarita Bajaj

INTRODUCTION

Vitamin D insufficiency remains a prevalent problem in the 21st century. Its deficiency is often clinically unrecognized; however, measurements in laboratory are easy to perform and treatment expenditure is also minimal. Vitamin D deficiency is plausibly implicated in several adverse health outcomes, including mortality, malignancies, cardiovascular diseases, immune intolerance, and blood glucose metabolism.[1] This problem becomes prominent amongst pregnant women, where the functions of vitamin D appear to be diverse and complex. Pregnant women with light pigmented skin are at low risk of vitamin D deficiency when compared to women with darker skin pigmentation.

VITAMIN D METABOLISM IN PREGNANCY

Vitamin D2 and D3 are 25-hydroxylated in the liver to produce the major circulating vitamin D metabolite in blood, 25-hydroxy vitamin D3 [25(OH)D3], which undergoes further hydroxylation, mainly in the kidney, to form the steroid hormone 1-α,25-dihydroxy vitamin D3 [$1,25(OH)_2D3$]. This hormone binds to intracellular vitamin D receptors to control expression of vitamin D-regulated genes all across the genome via epigenetic mechanisms. During pregnancy, maternal vitamin D metabolism is altered to enable transfer of calcium across the placenta to enable fetal skeletal development. Extra calcium is obtained mainly from increased maternal intestinal calcium absorption, a vitamin D-dependent process, and increased renal hydroxylation. Transplacental transfer of calcium to the fetus is also facilitated by expression of all key mediators of vitamin D metabolism in the placenta. Hormones involved in fetal growth, such as insulin-like growth factor-1 (IGF-1) and human placental lactogen (HPL) may also play a synergistic role.[2,3]

In maternal vitamin D deficiency, the maternal skeleton is also used as a source of calcium for the developing fetus. This process is mediated by parathyroid hormone (PTH), which mobilizes calcium in a vitamin D-independent mechanism. Further adaptations occur involving maternal PTH, parathyroid hormone-related protein (PTHrP), and interactions of prolactin, estradiol, and some other hormones during breastfeeding after the loss of placental influence on vitamin D metabolism.[4] Significant calcium losses are seen in lactating women, because of these calcium mobilizing processes. As little vitamin D is contained in breast milk, neonatal vitamin D deficiency may be worsened during lactation in deficient mothers, if supplementation is not provided to the neonate or insufficient amount is provided to the lactating mother.[5]

IMPACT OF VITAMIN D DEFICIENCY ON MATERNAL AND INFANT HEALTH

A number of fetal, neonatal, and maternal health problems have been associated with maternal vitamin D deficiency (Table 9-1).[6] In the mother, infertility, a lower success rate of *in vitro* fertilization (IVF), spontaneous preterm birth, an increased rate of cesarean section, preeclampsia, gestational diabetes mellitus (GDM), maternal osteomalacia, and muscle weakness have been described.[1] In the child, fetal growth retardation, neonatal hypocalcemia and seizures, and skeletal disorders, including rickets and osteopenia may be observed. Type 1 diabetes, effects on immune functioning, asthma, atopy, neurological diseases, an increased risk of human immunodeficiency virus (HIV) transmission as well as schizophrenia are some other possible disease associations.[7,8]

TABLE 9-1

Effects of Vitamin D Deficiency on Maternal and Fetal Health	
Maternal	*Fetal/neonatal*
• Preeclampsia • Bacterial vaginosis • GDM • Spontaneous preterm birth • Increased Cesarean section rate • PCOS • Decreased IVF success • Osteomalacia and muscle weakness.	• SGA (decreased birth weight, decreased infant size) • Fetal skeletal disorders • Neonatal hypocalcemia and seizures • Asthma • Type 1 diabetes mellitus • Multiple sclerosis • Autism • Maternal-fetal HIV transfer • Schizophrenia.

PCOS, polycystic ovarian syndrome; IVF, *in vitro* fertilization; HIV, human immunodeficiency virus, GDM, gestational diabetes mellitus; SGA, small for gestational age.

PHYSIOLOGY OF VITAMIN D DURING PREGNANCY AND LACTATION

During pregnancy and lactation, maternal physiology is changed to facilitate the transfer of calcium to both the fetus and the neonate, respectively. The fetus requires approximately 30 g of calcium during development, majority of which is needed in the third trimester. Increase in PTHrP during pregnancy results in an increase in the synthesis of 1,25(OH)$_2$D3. The increase in 1,25(OH)$_2$D3 causes maternal PTH levels to drop.[9] Serum calcium remains normal despite increased PTH bioactivity, as calcium is transferred to the fetus and lost in the urine. In normal pregnancy, maternal 1,25(OH)$_2$D3 gradually increases from the first trimester to a peak of twofolds of the nonpregnancy level in the third trimester. Pregnancy does not affect the clearance of 1,25(OH)$_2$D3. Increased production as well as an increase in vitamin D binding protein results in the rise in maternal serum levels.[10] The increased synthesis is mainly due to elevated 1α-hydroxylase activity in the maternal kidney, with some input from the placenta, decidua, and fetal kidney. Fetal calcium levels are greater than maternal levels throughout gestation since there is active transport of calcium across the placenta. Vitamin D levels in the fetus are up to 20% lower than maternal, predisposing the neonate to hypocalcemia and rickets.[11] Vitamin D in breast milk correlates well with maternal vitamin D concentrations, so breastfed infants are at a risk of persistent vitamin D deficiency if the mother is deficient.

IMPLICATIONS OF VITAMIN D DEFICIENCY IN FEMALE REPRODUCTION

Vitamin D and Fertility

There has been a demonstrated seasonal distribution in human natural conception and birth rates, with summers being the season of highest conception rate with strong seasonal contrast in luminosity.[12] The ovary being a target organ for 1,25(OH)$_2$D3, increases the possibility that this active metabolite of vitamin D might play a role in the modulation of ovarian activity.[13] Results of human studies have been contradictory on the role of vitamin D on human fertility and reproduction, which merits further evaluation by longitudinal studies.[14]

Infertility Treatment

Vitamin D levels in the serum and follicular fluid of women undergoing IVF treatment have been shown to have a positive correlation with the success of the procedure – each nanomole increase in follicular fluid vitamin D increases the likelihood for achieving clinical pregnancy by 2.4%.[15] A higher rate of ovarian follicle formation is observed in women with polycystic ovarian syndrome (PCOS) treated with calcium and vitamin D supplementation in addition to metformin as compared to metformin alone over a period of 3 months.[16]

Vitamin D and Hypertensive Disorders in Pregnancy

Seasonal patterns in preeclampsia, with higher incidence in winter and a lower incidence in summer, imply a role for vitamin D and sunlight.[17] The hallmark of preeclampsia is marked changes in vitamin D and calcium metabolism as compared to normal pregnancies. Normotensive pregnant women have high 25(OH)D levels than women suffering from preeclampsia.[18,19]

How vitamin D deficiency might be involved in pathophysiologic processes that cause preeclampsia remains unclear.[20] The placenta itself expresses 1α-hydroxylase and, thus, produces the active metabolite $1,25(OH)_2D3$.[21] Whether this placental production of vitamin D is a major contributor to the maternal vitamin D status or has mainly paracrine functions, is a matter of controversy.[4] In syncytiotrophoblasts from preeclamptic pregnancies, the expression and activity of 1α-hydroxylase is limited, implying a significant role for vitamin D in the placenta.[22] Vitamin D is a key regulator of target genes associated with implantation, trophoblast invasion, and implantation tolerance.[23]

Vitamin D and Mode of Delivery

The need of a primary cesarean section has been demonstrated to have an inverse association with the status of vitamin D. Severely vitamin D deficient women with levels of 25(OH)D below 37.5 nmol/L delivered nearly 4 times as often by cesarean section than those with values more than 37.5 nmol/L.[24]

Vitamin D and Spontaneous Preterm Birth

Bacterial vaginosis, an alteration of the normal balance of vaginal flora with marked growth of anaerobic bacteria, causes release of prostaglandins, inflammatory cytokines, and phospholipase A.[25] A linear inverse dose-response association has been documented between maternal vitamin D status and the prevalence of bacterial vaginosis in early pregnancy.[26] Since vitamin D has immunomodulatory and anti-inflammatory properties, a protective role on risk of spontaneous preterm birth is to be expected. Vitamin D also regulates calcium release within the muscle cell which is responsible for myometrial contractility. Deficiency of vitamin D levels may, therefore, increase the frequency of spontaneous preterm labor.[27]

Vitamin D and Other Reproductive Outcomes

Vitamin D has a complex relation with fetal growth that may vary by genotype, race, and other variables. Breast milk is an ideal nutrient for a newborn but is insufficient to maintain its vitamin D levels within the required range, resulting in the need for vitamin D replacement in many nursing mothers or their infants.[14]

Vitamin D and Fetal Programming

Vitamin D induces over 3,000 genes, and many of them play a vital role in fetal growth and development.[28] Vitamin D may, therefore, be particularly relevant to the "developmental origins" or "fetal programming hypothesis", which states that environmental factors, such as vitamin D influence the genomic programming of fetal and neonatal development and subsequent disease risk in both childhood and later adult life.[29] Children of mothers with low vitamin D levels during gestation suffer more often from chronic diseases in later life.[30] The epigenetic mechanisms, which lead to persistent structural and functional changes in the endocrine system have been hypothesized.

Vitamin D and Other Pregnancy-associated Disorders

There is a correlation between low maternal vitamin D levels and GDM as might be expected from its association with insulin resistance (IR) and type 2 diabetes. The role played by confounding factors, such as ethnicity and obesity is not established.[1] One of the trials on supplementation with intravenous and oral 1,25$(OH)_2$D3 in 12 women with GDM showed no change in blood glucose but lowered insulin levels following replacement, implying an increase in insulin sensitivity.[31]

The prevalence of vitamin D deficiency in the nonpregnant HIV positive population has been variably quoted as between 30 and 50% and may influence disease progression and survival in these patients.[32] Vitamin D supplementation in HIV-infected pregnant women demonstrates a potentially beneficial effect of adequate vitamin D status on HIV disease and related outcomes.[33]

VITAMIN D SUPPLEMENTATION IN PREGNANCY

In the UK, national recommendations suggest that vitamin D supplementation of 400 IU/day during pregnancy should be given to prevent rickets. However, the guidelines differ between different advisory groups and countries.[34] The US-based Institute of Medicine (IOM) recommends a daily intake of 400–600 IU of vitamin D for all age groups (except the elderly), including pregnant and lactating women, and infants. Studies in nonpregnant individuals show that to achieve a significant change in serum 1,25$(OH)_2$D3 levels, large doses of supplemental vitamin D are required. Evidence for appropriate dosing of vitamin D supplementation in pregnancy above the current recommended 400 IU/day dose is awaited. It is hoped that data will come from randomized control trials that have been adequately designed to identify the potential direct benefit of high-dose supplementation to maternal and fetal outcomes.

It will develop an understanding of whom to treat, along with the role of biochemical screening for vitamin D deficiency in pregnancy.

Despite an increasing awareness of possible links between vitamin D deficiency and disease, there is a lack of evidence for causality over association. Women continue to remain deficient in vitamin D during pregnancy despite supplementation guidance.[35]

The most potent, best-tolerated, and effective route of administration is oral supplementation. Optimal levels of 1,25$(OH)_2$D3 for the non-classical actions of vitamin D in the reproductive period are yet to be established. Whether vitamin D supplementation started preconceptionally is protective against preeclampsia and other adverse pregnancy outcomes also remains unclear. Clinicians should, however, ensure the widespread uptake of recommended supplementation and aim towards strategies to improve the access to supplements that are cheap and palatable for pregnant women.

Pregnant women should undoubtedly consume 5–10 times more supplementation of vitamin D than that has been recommended in the last few decades.[14] Recommendations are awaited from organizations involved in women's health care, such as the World Health Organization (WHO) and the International Federation of Gynecology and Obstetrics (FIGO), that focus primarily on pregnant and lactating women in order to exhaust the possibilities for the health of mother and child, as per the epidemic status of hypovitaminosis.[36]

CONCLUSION

Vitamin D deficiency during pregnancy and lactation mostly goes unrecognized, but it may produce various maternal, fetal, and neonatal health problems. There is a need for high quality, large scale randomized control trials for determining the appropriate levels of 1,25$(OH)_2$D3 in the reproductive years of women and during pregnancy especially, so as to benefit the mother and the fetus adequately.

REFERENCES

1. Barrett H, McElduff A. Vitamin D and pregnancy: An old problem revisited. *Best Pract Res Clin Endocrinol Metab*. 2010;24:527-53.
2. Shin JS, Choi MY, Longtine MS, Nelson DM. Vitamin D effects on pregnancy and the placenta. *Placenta*. 2010;31:1027-34.
3. Stephanou A, Ross R, Handwerger S. Regulation of human placental lactogen expression by 1,25-dihydroxyvitamin D3. *Endocrinology*. 1994;135:2651-6.
4. Kovacs CS. Vitamin D in pregnancy and lactation: maternal, fetal, and neonatal outcomes from human and animal studies. *Am J Clin Nutr*. 2008;88:520S-8S.
5. Hollis BW, Wagner CL. Assessment of dietary vitamin D requirements during pregnancy and lactation. *Am J Clin Nutr*. 2004;79:717-26.
6. Liu NQ, Hewison M. Vitamin D, the placenta and pregnancy. *Arch Biochem Biophys*. 2011.

7. Radhika AG, Goel M, Radhakrishnan G, Arora S, Guleria K. Severe osteomalacia presenting as numerous fractures in late pregnancy. *Int J Gynecol Obstet.* 2008;100:92-3.
8. Fernández-Alonso AM, Dionis-Sánchez EC, Chedraui P, González-Salmerón MD, Pérez-López FR; Spanish Vitamin D and Women's Health Research Group. First trimester maternal serum 25-hydroxyvitamin D status and pregnancy outcome. *Int J Gynecol Obstet.* 2012;116:6-9.
9. Kovacs CS, Kronenberg HM. Maternal-fetal calcium and bone metabolism during pregnancy, puerperium, and lactation. *Endocr Rev.* 1997;18:832-72.
10. Bouillon R, Van Assche FA, Van Baelen H, Heyns W, De Moor P. Influence of the vitamin D-binding protein on the serum concentration of 1,25-dihydroxyvitamin D3. Significance of the free 1,25-dihydroxyvitamin D3 concentration. *J Clin Invest.* 1981;67:589-96.
11. Morley R, Carlin JB, Pasco JA, Wark JD. Maternal 25-hydroxyvitamin D and parathyroid hormone concentrations and offspring birth size. *J Clin Endocrinol Metab.* 2006;91:906-12.
12. Rojansky N, Brzezinski A, Schenker JG. Seasonality in human reproduction: an update. *Hum Reprod.* 1992;7:735-45.
13. Dokoh S, Donaldson CA, Marion SL, Pike JW, Haussler MR. The ovary: a target organ for 1,25-dihydroxyvitamin D3. *Endocrinology.* 1983;112:200-6.
14. Grundmann M, von Versen-Höynck F. Vitamin D – roles in women's reproductive health? *Reprod Biol Endocrinol.* 2011;9:146.
15. Ozkan S, Jindal S, Greenseid K, Shu J, Zeitlian G, Hickman C, et al. Replete vitamin D stores predict reproductive success following in vitro fertilization. *Fertil Steril.* 2010;94:1314-9.
16. Rashidi B, Haghollahi F, Shariat M, Zayerii F. The effects of calcium-vitamin D and metformin on polycystic ovary syndrome: a pilot study. *Taiwan J Obstet Gynecol.* 2009;48: 142-7.
17. TePoel MR, Saftlas AF, Wallis AB. Association of seasonality with hypertension in pregnancy: a systematic review. *J Reprod Immunol.* 2011;89:140-52.
18. Bodnar LM, Catov JM, Simhan HN, Holick MF, Powers RW, Roberts JM. Maternal vitamin D deficiency increases the risk of preeclampsia. *J Clin Endocrinol Metab.* 2007;92:3517-22.
19. Robinson CJ, Alanis MC, Wagner CL, Hollis BW, Johnson DD. Plasma 25- hydroxyvitamin D levels in early-onset severe preeclampsia. *Am J Obstet Gynecol.* 2010;203:366.
20. Liu NQ, Kaplan AT, Lagishetty V, Ouyang YB, Ouyang Y, Simmons CF, et al. Vitamin D and the regulation of placental inflammation. *J Immunol.* 2011;186:5968-74.
21. Barrera D, Avila E, Hernandez G, Mendez I, Gonzalez L, Halhali A, et al. Calcitriol affects hCG gene transcription in cultured human syncytiotrophoblasts. *Reprod Biol Endocrinol.* 2008;6:3.
22. Diaz L, Arranz C, Avila E, Halhali A, Vilchis F, Larrea F. Expression and activity of 25-hydroxyvitamin D-1 alpha-hydroxylase are restricted in cultures of human syncytiotrophoblast cells from preeclamptic pregnancies. *J Clin Endocrinol Metab.* 2002;87:3876-82.
23. Evans KN, Bulmer JN, Kilby MD, Hewison M. Vitamin D and placental-decidual function. *J Soc Gynecol Investig.* 2004;11:263-71.
24. Merewood A, Mehta SD, Chen TC, Bauchner H, Holick MF. Association between vitamin D deficiency and primary cesarean section. *J Clin Endocrinol Metab.* 2009;94:940-5.
25. Allsworth JE, Peipert JF. Prevalence of bacterial vaginosis: 2001-2004 National Health and Nutrition Examination Survey data. *Obstet Gynecol.* 2007;109:114-20.

26. Bodnar LM, Krohn MA, Simhan HN. Maternal vitamin D deficiency is associated with bacterial vaginosis in the first trimester of pregnancy. *J Nutr.* 2009;139:1157-61.
27. Chesney RW. Vitamin D and The Magic Mountain: the anti-infectious role of the vitamin. *J Pediatr.* 2010;156:698-703.
28. Kho AT, Bhattacharya S, Tantisira KG, Carey VJ, Gaedigk R, Leeder JS, et al. Transcriptomic analysis of human lung development. *Am J Respir Crit Care Med.* 2010;181:54-63.
29. Erkkola M, Kaila M, Nwaru BI, Kronberg-Kippila C, Ahonen S, Nevalainen J, et al. Maternal vitamin D intake during pregnancy is inversely associated with asthma and allergic rhinitis in 5-year-old children. *Clin Exp Allergy.* 2009;39:875-82.
30. Altschuler EL. Low maternal vitamin D and schizophrenia in offspring. *Lancet.* 2001; 358:1464.
31. Rudnicki PM, Molsted-Pedersen L. Effect of 1,25-dihydroxycholecalciferol on glucose metabolism in gestational diabetes mellitus. *Diabetologia.* 1997;40:40-4.
32. Villamor E. A potential role for vitamin D on HIV infection? *Nutr Rev.* 2006;64:226-33.
33. Mehta S, Giovannucci E, Mugusi FM, Spiegelman D, Aboud S, Hertzmark E, et al. Vitamin D status of HIV-infected women and its associations with HIV disease progression, anemia, and mortality. *PLoS One.* 2010;50:e8770.
34. Hypponen E, Boucher BJ. Avoidance of vitamin D deficiency in pregnancy in the United Kingdom: the case for a unified approach in National policy. *Br J Nutr.* 2010;104:309-14.
35. Finer S, Khan KS, Hitman GA, Griffiths C, Martineau A, Meads C. *ACTA Obstet Gynecol.* 2012;91:59-163.
36. Pérez-López FR. Low maternal vitamin D status during pregnancy requires appropriate therapeutic intervention. *Inter J Gynecol Obstet.* 2012;116:4-5.

10

Bone Disorders and Pregnancy

Sarita Bajaj, Afreen Khan

INTRODUCTION

Calcium homeostasis is maintained mainly by the intricate interrelationship between parathyroid hormone (PTH) and vitamin D in the nonpregnant state. Pregnancy and lactation dramatically alter the calcium metabolism. A significant demand is imposed by the developing fetus on maternal calcium homeostasis. About 25–30 g calcium, equivalent to 2–3% of the total body calcium content of the mother is transferred to the fetus during pregnancy. The second and third trimesters are the periods when maximum transfer of calcium takes place, and fetal bone development is reaching peak. Approximately 200 mg of calcium is deposited during the third trimester in the fetal skeleton per day.[1] The mother further loses 300–400 mg calcium daily in the breast milk, if pregnancy is followed by a period of breastfeeding. Studies have demonstrated 2–9% lower bone mineral density (BMD) in postpartum women than in matched controls, in spite of endocrine changes that induce compensatory mechanisms to counteract the calcium loss. A further 1–6% loss in maternal BMD is associated with breastfeeding period of 6 months and pregnancy-related osteoporosis has been reported. These factors raise the possibility of low BMD and bone disorders in multiple pregnancies and prolonged breastfeeding, especially in developing countries.[2]

CALCIUM METABOLISM DURING PREGNANCY

Calcium

In pregnancy, calcium homeostasis differs slightly from that of the nonpregnant state in order to meet the calcium demands of the mother and fetus (Figure 10-1).

About 30 g of calcium is accreted by the developing fetal skeleton by term; out of which, 80% occur during the third trimester. The maternal intestinal calcium absorption

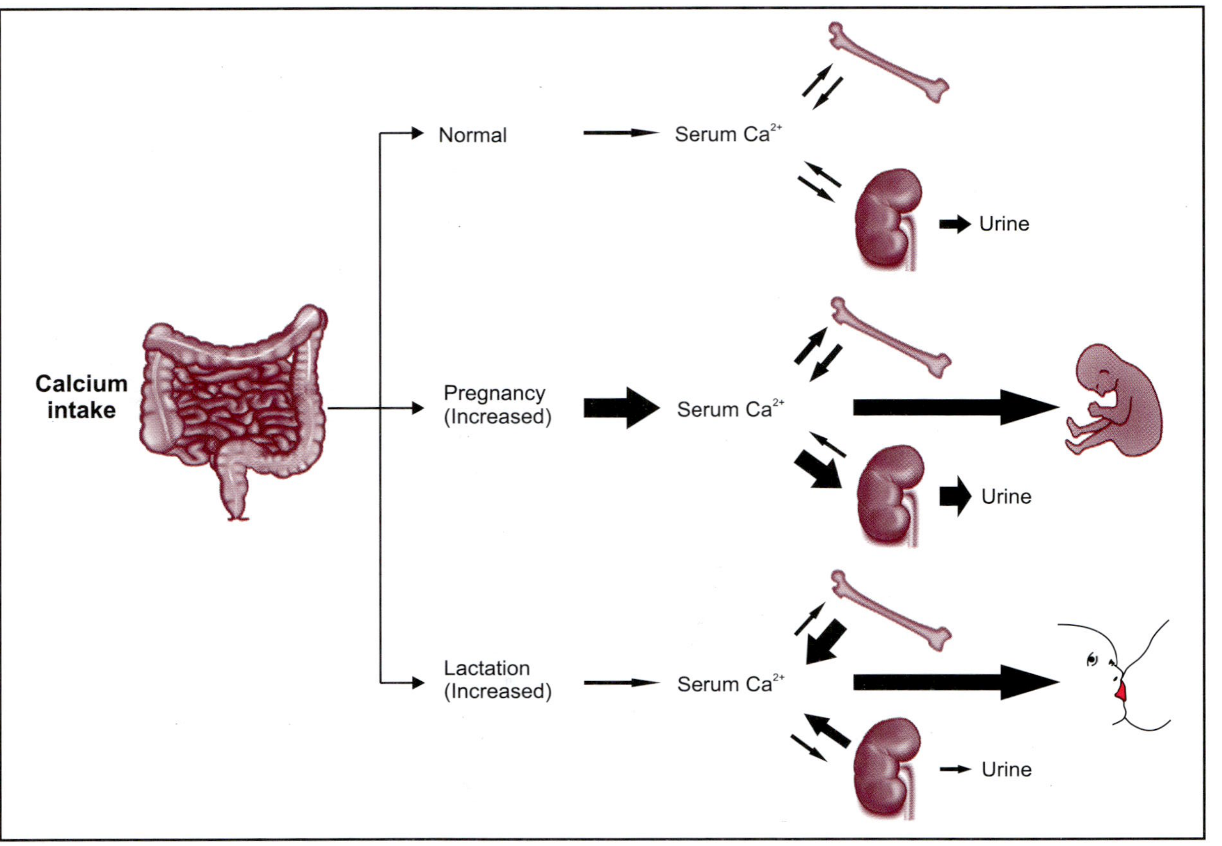

Figure 10-1 Calcium homeostasis in human pregnancy and lactation compared with normal. The thickness of arrows indicates a relative increase or decrease with respect to the normal and nonpregnant state. *Adapted from* Kovacs CS, Kronenberg HM. Maternal-fetal calcium and bone metabolism during pregnancy, puerperium and lactation. *Endocr Rev*. 1997;18:832-72.

is doubled, mediated by 1,25-dihydroxyvitamin D3 [1,25$(OH)_2$D3] or calcitriol and other factors meet this demand for calcium. The ionized calcium (the physiologically important fraction of calcium), however, remains constant throughout pregnancy. The total serum calcium (sum of the ionized, complexed, and albumin-bound fractions of calcium in the circulation) in contrast, decreases in pregnancy as a result of decline in serum albumin.[3]

Vitamin D

Studies in pregnant women have shown that increased kidney 1α-hydroxylase and the placental expression of 1α-hydroxylase, which enhances maternal intestinal calcium absorption, result in a 2 times increase in the levels of 1,25$(OH)_2$D3 during pregnancy.[4]

Parathyroid Hormone-related Peptide

Parathyroid hormone-related peptide (PTHrP) is another calciotropic hormone known to increase during pregnancy. Its levels remain elevated during lactation to provide sufficient calcium for breast milk production. The calcium levels are increased by skeletal mobilization.[4]

Parathyroid Hormone

Plasma PTH levels fall during the first trimester but progressively rise throughout the remainder of pregnancy. Lower calcium concentration in pregnant woman likely results in its increased levels. Increased plasma volume, increased glomerular filtration rate (GFR), and maternal-fetal transfer of calcium are the likely causes of low calcium levels. Another mechanism that increases PTH during pregnancy is the effect of estrogen, which appears to block the action of PTH on bone resorption. A physiological hyperparathyroidism of pregnancy, thus, occurs as a result of these actions and is likely to supply the fetus with adequate calcium.[5]

Calcitonin

Calcitonin levels during pregnancy and lactation are markedly higher than in the nonpregnant state since these are the periods of profound calcium stress.[6]

CALCIUM METABOLISM DURING LACTATION

Calcium

A daily loss of about 280–400 mg of calcium occurs through breast milk. These losses can reach up to 1000 mg or more in women who are nursing twins. The main mechanism by which lactating women appear to meet these calcium requirements is a temporary demineralization of the skeleton. This demineralization seems to be mediated by PTHrP in the setting of a decrease in estrogen levels rather than by PTH or calcitriol. However, there is an increase in the mean ionized calcium levels of exclusively lactating women, although it remains within the normal limits.[3]

Parathyroid Hormone-related Peptide

During lactation, PTHrP produced by the mammary tissue combines with low estradiol (and possibly other factors) to stimulate osteoclast-mediated bone resorption.[7]

Vitamin D

In lactating women, vitamin D levels normally fall to prepregnancy values, and intestinal calcium absorption also normalizes. This shows that lactation may not require a normal vitamin D endocrine system in transferring calcium to breast milk.[7]

Parathyroid Hormone

During lactation, 'intact' PTH has been found to be decreased by 50% or more in the first several months. At weaning, it increases to normal, but after weaning, it may rise above normal.[3]

Calcitonin

In the first 6 weeks of lactation, calcitonin levels are increased. In the short-term, calcitonin is needed to prevent severe losses of mineral content and potential skeletal fragility. However, as the skeletal losses of mineral are restored anyway, it is not required in the long-term.[3]

BONE CHANGES IN PREGNANCY AND LACTATION

The changes in BMD during pregnancy have been studied utilizing different methods of assessment, including quantitative ultrasound and radiology. Dual-energy X-ray absorptiometry (DXA) has been used by most investigators to investigate pregnancy-related alterations in areal bone mineral density (aBMD). The prepregnant to early postpartum period and early pregnancy to late pregnancy phases demonstrate a progressive fall in BMD. The actual pathophysiology involved in BMD changes in pregnancy is still largely unknown, although factors that influence these changes have been studied in various settings.[8]

While some studies suggest a decrease in bone density in skeletal regions, such as the spine and hip, which are rich in trabecular bone with no change or an increase in regions rich in cortical bone, other studies have not shown this pattern. For reasons which are unclear, a considerable variation between women in the skeletal response to pregnancy has been suggested by many studies. The magnitude of skeletal response in pregnancy may be influenced by disparities in mechanical loading resulting from differences in maternal body weight and weight gain. The calcium intake of the mother before or during pregnancy may also influence the amount of skeletal calcium mobilized. Other factors, such as aging, body weight, and calcium intake, which may have influence on the maternal skeleton independent of pregnancy, have not been considered by most studies.[9]

Maternal BMD decreases on an average by 5% during pregnancy and breastfeeding despite the body's attempts to maintain calcium homeostasis. The rate of loss of BMD by 1–3% per year that occurs in women with postmenopausal osteoporosis is far exceeded by the peak rate of loss of 1–3% per month during pregnancy and lactation. The regulation of maternal BMD, however, is also affected by the nutritional intake; which is often higher in pregnant and lactating women than other women as well as changes in the level of physical activity. Additionally, the bone loss associated with pregnancy and breastfeeding is usually recovered after weaning as demonstrated by longitudinal studies.[2] No significant reduction in bone loss is seen with calcium supplementation during lactation. It seems certain that any acute changes in bone metabolism during pregnancy do not normally cause long-term changes in skeletal calcium content or strength.[3]

DISORDERS OF BONE METABOLISM

The differing hormonal changes that occur in pregnancy and lactation as compared to the nonpregnant state influence the disorders of bone and mineral homeostasis in these two reproductive periods.

Primary Hyperparathyroidism

Primary hyperparathyroidism is a rare occurrence during pregnancy with a prevalence of 0.5–1.4%.[10] More than two-thirds of the cases are associated with significant morbidity to the fetus and mother. Increased rate of abortions, severe intrauterine growth retardation (IUGR), and stillbirth are the adverse fetal outcomes associated with hyperparathyroidism. The calcium levels drop precipitously in the neonate once the cord is clamped after delivery due to suppression of the fetal parathyroids during pregnancy in hyperparathyroidism. These suppressed parathyroids are unable to respond well. The net result is severe hypocalcemic tetany and seizures that require prolonged neonatal care. On the other hand, neonatal hypocalcemia may be the only sign that may detect mild-to-moderately severe hyperparathyroidism in the mother.[11]

Primary hyperparathyroidism during pregnancy may result in maternal complications like nephrolithiasis, hyperemesis, or even severe hypercalcemic crisis that may be life threatening. Pregnancy normally results in decreased maternal serum calcium levels secondary to increased calcium demands. Hence, hypercalcemia, the most prevalent laboratory finding in primary hyperparathyroidism may not be seen in cases of hyperparathyroidism during pregnancy, making the diagnosis challenging and increasing the risk of complications.[10]

During the first trimester of pregnancy, if symptoms and calcium levels are controlled by drugs, medical treatment may be an option. However, oral phosphates are classified into pregnancy class C drugs. Furthermore, usage of bisphosphonates (BSP) is indicated as short-term treatment in cases of severe hypercalcemia, despite the fact that they have recently been used without detrimental effects on both mother and fetus. Hence, hydration, calcitonin, intravenous magnesium, or the recently mentioned usage of cinacalset are the only preferable medication options available. Surgical treatment in the third trimester, on the other hand, has shown to be associated with high complication rates. Thus, it might be best to continue conservative management until postpartum, if symptoms and serum calcium levels are well controlled. However, if symptoms persist and calcium levels remain above 11 mg/dL, surgical treatment is indicated regardless of the trimester of pregnancy.[10]

Hypoparathyroidism in Pregnancy

Hypoparathyroidism may not uncommonly be encountered as a preexisting condition during pregnancy. Low calcium levels, seen normally during normal pregnancy, may pose a great challenge in diagnosing hypoparathyroidism for the first time in pregnancy. However, levels of ionized calcium may help in confirming the diagnosis, since its levels remain normal during pregnancy. Maintenance of near normal calcium in the mother is the principle of management of hypoparathyroidism during pregnancy in order to prevent fetal hyperparathyroidism, which has serious consequences, including fetal death.[3] The requirement of calcitriol and calcium may come down during the latter half of pregnancy and even more during lactation in a patient on treatment for hypoparathyroidism due to the effects of PTHrP. This makes it mandatory to closely monitor calcium levels to titrate the dosage so that adverse fetal consequences may be prevented. Hypercalcemia may result from inadvertent excessive use of calcitriol.[11]

Pseudohypoparathyroidism

Pseudohypoparathyroidism is a state characterized by inherited resistance to PTH resulting in hypocalcemia, hypophosphatemia, and high PTH levels. However, calcium levels have been reported to become normal in these patients during pregnancy without ingesting therapeutic amounts of calcium and vitamin D, the mechanism of which is still unclear.[3] The requirements of calcitriol and calcium have been reported to be variable. Increased generation from non-PTH/PTHrP-dependent sources like placenta seems to reduce calcitriol requirement in some cases. Maintenance of maternal serum calcium levels is the principle of management in these patients, as maternal hypocalcemia may cause fetal hyperparathyroidism. Since the placental source of 1,25(OH)$_2$D3 is lost during lactation, and pseudohypoparathyroidism is associated with resistance to renal action of PTHrP, the dosage of calcium and calcitriol usually reverts to prepregnant levels.[11]

Osteoporosis in Pregnancy

Transient osteoporosis, first reported 50 years ago in the hip in the last trimester of pregnancy, is an idiopathic condition characterized by swelling in the lower limbs and attacks of periarticular pain associated with development of localized osteoporosis in the subjacent periarticular bone. However, it may also affect middle-aged men and nonpregnant women. The knees or talus have been reported to be affected. Clinical manifestations, which may last up to 1 year, adversely affect the quality of life and insufficiency fractures may be a complication; however, complete recovery is the rule.[12]

According to a case report published by Willis-Owen et al.,[13] a 34-year old Persian woman presented at 22 weeks of pregnancy with a 2 weeks history of left hip pain with no apparent precipitating event. She had no history of smoking or alcohol, no history of corticosteroids, anticonvulsant, or anticoagulant use, and she was not on any other medications. With time, her hip pain worsened and the patient started to experience pain in the contralateral hip as well. Imaging of her hips was avoided, because of her pregnancy. By 36 weeks of pregnancy, the patient was unable to bear weight and became wheelchair bound. She was brought to the attention of the orthopedic team. Plain radiographs following delivery revealed a displaced intracapsular femoral neck fracture on the left and a valgus impacted right intracapsular femoral neck fracture on the right. The radiographs also revealed considerable osteopenia. Magnetic resonance imaging (MRI) revealed these fractures with reduced signal on T1 and increased signal on T2 in the femoral necks, thus, establishing the diagnosis of transient osteoporosis of pregnancy.[13]

Preconceptional osteoporosis and increased bone turnover in pregnancy and lactation may also result in fragility fractures in pregnancy and the puerperium. Drugs like heparin, corticosteroids, and anticonvulsants when used for long-term may cause secondary osteoporosis. Excessive skeletal calcium resorption may result from low dietary intake of calcium and vitamin D. Hence, adequate calcium and vitamin D intake and exercise should be instituted when needed. Possible adverse effects on the developing fetus contraindicate the use of specific treatment like bisphosphonates or calcitonin.

Radiographs are not useful for demonstrating early osteopenia and are avoided in pregnancy wherever possible. MRI reveals low signal intensity of bone marrow on T1 weighted images and high signal on T2 weighted images are suggestive of bone marrow edema. Symptoms resolve naturally over the course of 3–6 months.[13]

CONCLUSION

Novel regulatory systems specific to pregnancy and lactation complement the usual regulators of calcium homeostasis. In order to meet the fetal demand for calcium, intestinal absorption of calcium increases 2 times as compared to early in pregnancy. On the other hand, during lactation, skeletal resorption of calcium is the dominant mechanism by which calcium is supplied to the breast milk along with renal calcium conservation. It is clear from observational studies and clinical trials that calcium supplementation has little or no impact on the amount of bone loss during lactation, although its supplementation during pregnancy enables the mother to increase its absorption. Through mechanisms that remain unclear, the skeleton promptly recovers to achieve the prepregnancy bone mass from that during lactation. Although in some women the transient loss of bone mass during lactation can compromise skeletal strength and lead to fragility fractures, the majority of women can be assured that the changes in calcium and bone metabolism during pregnancy and lactation are normal, healthy, and without adverse consequences in the long-term.

REFERENCES

1. Pitkin RM. Calcium metabolism in pregnancy and the perinatal period: A review. *Am J Obstet Gynecol.* 1985;151:99-109.
2. Lenora J, Lekamwasam S, Karlsson MK. Effects of multiparity and prolonged breast-feeding on maternal bone mineral density: a community-based cross-sectional study. *BMC Womens Health.* 2009;9:19.
3. Kovacs CS, Fuleihan Gel-H. Calcium and bone disorders during pregnancy and lactation. *Endocrinol Metab Clin North Am.* 2006;35:21-51.
4. Tangpricha V. Maternal hypoparathyroidism due to an activating mutation of the calcium sensing receptor during pregnancy and lactation. *Endocr Pract.* 2012:1-5.
5. Pitkin RM, Reynolds WA, Williams GA, Hargis GK. Calcium metabolism in normal pregnancy: a longitudinal study. *Am J Obstet Gynecol.* 1979;133:781-90.
6. Weiss M, Eisenstein Z, Ramot Y, Piptz S, Shulman A, Frenkel Y. Renal reabsorption of inorganic phosphorus in pregnancy in relation to the calciotropic hormones. *Br J Obstet Gynaecol.* 1998;105:195-9.
7. Fudge NJ, Kovacs CS. Pregnancy up-regulates intestinal calcium absorption and skeletal mineralization independently of the vitamin D receptor. *Endocrinology.* 2010;151: 886-95.
8. To WW, Wong MW. Bone mineral density changes in pregnancies with gestational hypertension: a longitudinal study using quantitative ultrasound measurements. *Arch Gynecol Obstet.* 2011;284:39-44.
9. Olausson H, Laskey MA, Goldberg GR, Prentice A. Changes in bone mineral status and bone size during pregnancy, and the influences of body weight and calcium intake. *Am J Clin Nutr.* 2008;88:1032-9.

10. Petousis S, Kourtis A, Anastasilakis CD, Makedou K, Giomisi A, Kalogiannidis I, et al. Successful surgical treatment of primary hyperparathyroidism during the third trimester of pregnancy. *J Musculoskelet Neuronal Interact*. 2012;12:43-5.
11. Mahadevan S, Kumaravel V, Bharath R. Calcium and bone disorders in pregnancy. Indian. *J Endocrinol Metab*. 2012;16:358-63.
12. Rozenbaum M, Boulman N, Rimar D, Kaly L, Rosner I and Slobodin G. Uncommon Transient Osteoporosis of Pregnancy at Multiple Sites Associated with Cytomegalovirus Infection: Is There a Link? *IMAJ*. 2011;13:709-11.
13. Willis-Owen CA, Daurka JS, Chen A and Lewis A. Bilateral femoral neck fractures due to transient osteoporosis of pregnancy: a case report. *Cases J*. 2008;1:120.

11

Pituitary Disorders in Pregnancy

Simon Rajaratnam, Geeta Chacko

INTRODUCTION

The pituitary gland (Figure 11-1) increases in size during pregnancy due to lactotroph hyperplasia and hypertrophy. Following delivery, the gland gradually returns to its normal size.[1] Due to normal physiological changes, the assessment of pituitary functions differs from that of the nonpregnant state.

PHYSIOLOGICAL CHANGES OF THE PITUITARY HORMONE AXES DURING PREGNANCY

The normal physiologic changes include lactotroph hypertrophy, progressive increase in serum prolactin (PRL) levels, production of placental variant of growth hormone (GH-V), increase in corticotropin releasing hormone (CRH) – mainly from the

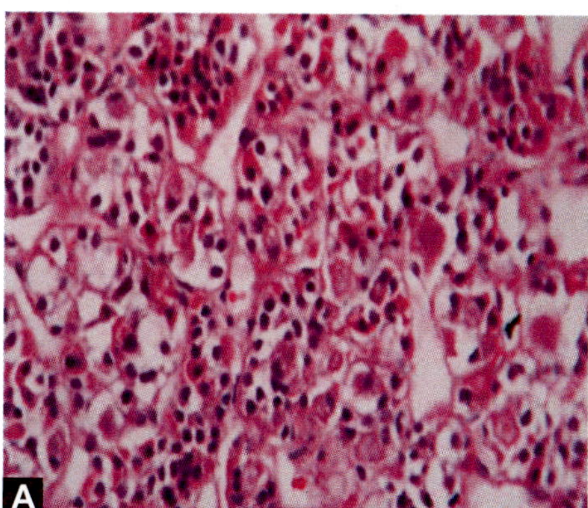

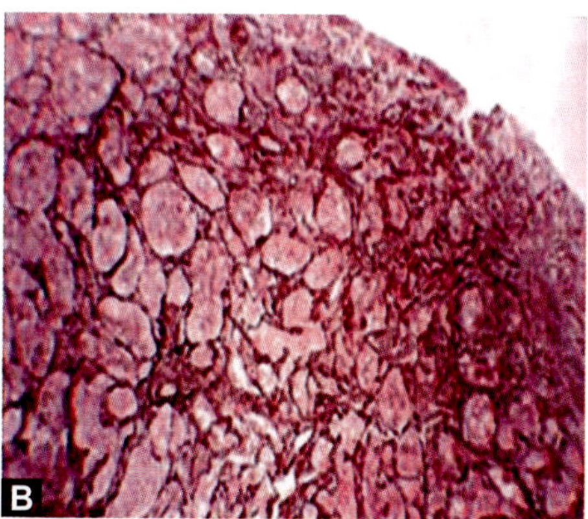

Figure 11-1 Pituitary gland. **A,** Normal histology. **B,** Normal acinar structure seen with reticulin stain.

placenta, decline in thyroid-stimulating hormone (TSH) in the first trimester due to the effect of human chorionic gonadotropin (hCG), and increased clearance of vasopressin due to placental vasopressinase.[2]

Growth Hormone

During pregnancy, pituitary growth hormone (GH) levels decrease and GH-V levels increase and peak by the third trimester of pregnancy. The actions of GH-V are similar to GH, but it has less lactogenic activity.[3]

Hypothalamic-pituitary-adrenal Axis

Placental CRH stimulates the production of adrenocorticotropic hormone (ACTH), both from placenta and maternal pituitary gland. Placental CRH is required for fetal adrenal development and for determining the onset of labor.[4] Cortisol levels progressively increase during pregnancy, and there is a final surge during labor. Cortisol binding globulin levels also increase during pregnancy. The normal circadian rhythm of cortisol is preserved. Placental 11β-hydroxysteroid dehydrogenase type 2 (11β-HSD2) protects the fetus from the effects of excess maternal cortisol (Figure 11-2).

Prolactin Axis

Estrogen and progesterone stimulation leads to progressive increase in serum PRL levels during pregnancy.

TRH–TSH Axis

Although the appearance and distribution of thyrotropic cells and thyrotropin-releasing hormone (TRH) are preserved, there is decreased production of maternal TSH in the first trimester of pregnancy due to its biochemical similarity to hCG. TSH levels return to normal in the second and third trimesters of pregnancy. In twin pregnancies and molar pregnancies, there occurs a greater lowering of maternal TSH levels.

During pregnancy, there is increased production of thyroxine-binding globulin (TBG), and this leads to increased levels of total thyroid hormone. Placental type II deiodinase converts thyroxine (T_4) to triiodothyronine (T_3) and maintains local T_3 production. Placental deiodination is responsible for increased T_4 requirement throughout pregnancy.[3] Low maternal T_4 levels in the second trimester lead to permanent neurological deficits in the developing fetus.[5,6]

The fetal hypothalamic-pituitary portal circulation is functional by 10–12 weeks of gestation and active iodine trapping can be detected by 12 weeks of gestation. Placental deiodination protects the fetus from excess maternal T_4.

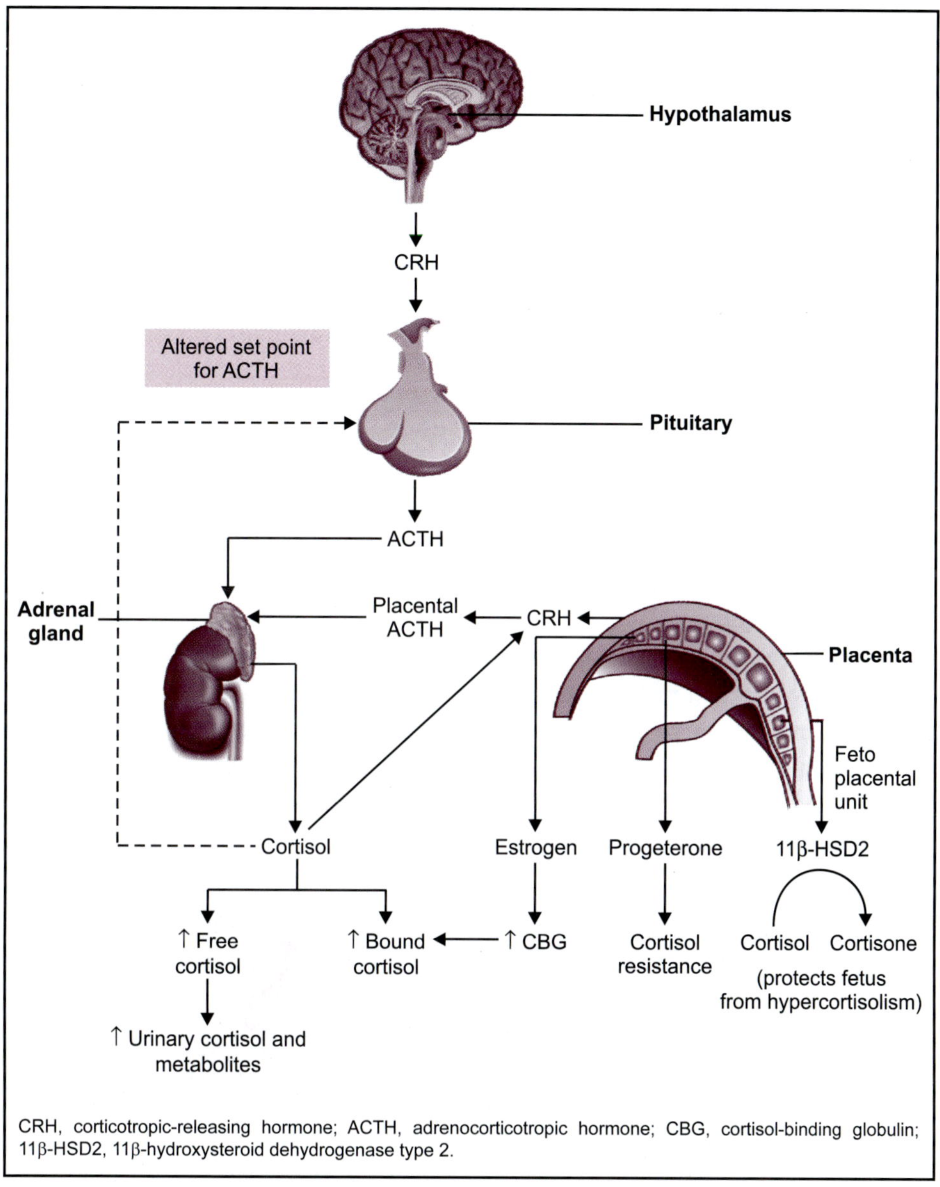

CRH, corticotropic-releasing hormone; ACTH, adrenocorticotropic hormone; CBG, cortisol-binding globulin; 11β-HSD2, 11β-hydroxysteroid dehydrogenase type 2.

Figure 11-2 Physiological changes in hypothalamic-pituitary-adrenal axis during pregnancy.

Gonadotropin Axis

As a result of placental sex steroid production, pituitary gonadotropins [follicle stimulating hormone (FSH) and luteinizing hormone (LH)] levels decline and become undetectable by the second trimester of pregnancy.

Renin-angiotensin-aldosterone System

Renin activity peaks towards the end of the first trimester of pregnancy and then declines in the third trimester of pregnancy. As a result, aldosterone levels reach values that are 5–8 times higher than that of the nonpregnant state.[2]

Posterior Pituitary

Placental vasopressinase is associated with increased vasopressin (AVP) degradation, and this may unmask borderline diabetes insipidus or worsen it during pregnancy.

ANTERIOR PITUITARY DISORDERS

Acromegaly

Excess of GH is usually associated with impaired fertility. In women with acromegaly (Figure 11-3), the occurrence of pregnancy can be associated with complications due to tumor expansion, excess GH and insulin-like growth factor-1 (IGF-1), and those related to treatment.[7]

Several factors may impact the course of pregnancy in acromegaly. GH does not cross the placenta, and maternal GH excess does not interfere with the growth of the fetus. Impaired pituitary function can, however, lead to spontaneous abortion. These women are also prone to associated medical problems like impaired glucose tolerance, diabetes, and hypertension. They are also at an increased risk for cardiomyopathy and coronary artery disease. During pregnancy, the normal pituitary gland increases in size

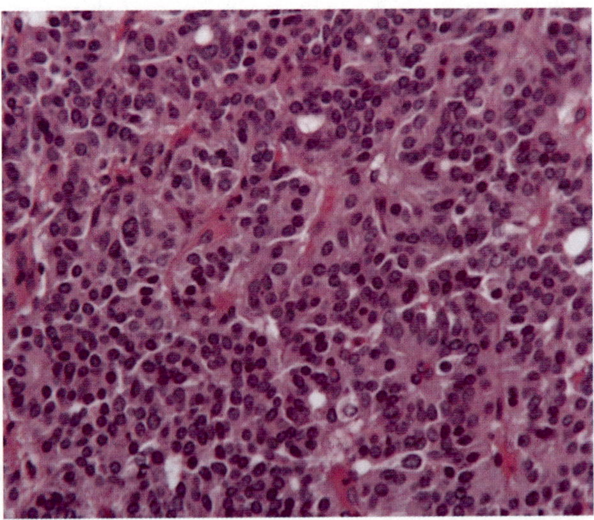

Figure 11-3 Pituitary adenoma.

and an increase in the size of these tumors during pregnancy can impair vision due to compression of the optic chiasm. There is also an increased risk of hemorrhage due to the enhanced vascularity of these tumors.[8]

Conventional radioimmunoassays cannot distinguish pituitary GH from GH-V. The oral glucose tolerance test (OGTT) is not well established for the diagnosis of acromegaly in pregnancy. IGF-1 levels which are elevated in both normal and acromegalic pregnancies are not useful for diagnosis. TRH causes paradoxical GH release in patients with acromegaly, which does not occur with the placental variant. Pituitary GH is released in a pulsatile manner, whereas GH-V is not.[9] GH-V levels become undetectable within 24 hours following delivery.

An MRI scan can identify more than 95% of tumors in these patients.

Bromocriptine has been used for the treatment of acromegaly during pregnancy. There is not much experience with cabergoline. Octreotide crosses the placenta and can affect the developing fetus. Pegvisomant has been tried in one patient with acromegaly in pregnancy. If tumor expansion occurs despite medical treatment, these patients should undergo transsphenoidal surgery.[3]

TSH Adenomas

Three cases of TSH adenomas in pregnancy have been reported. Hyperthyroidism in these patients was controlled with octreotide and antithyroid medication.[3]

Prolactinomas

Microprolactinomas (<10 mm) and macroprolactinomas (>10 mm) are associated with gonadal dysfunction and infertility. They respond to dopamine agonists like bromocriptine and cabergoline.[10] These patients may also require clomiphene and hCG rarely to induce ovulation.[11]

Prolactin levels 100–200 μg/L are diagnostic of prolactinomas; however, a prolactinoma cannot be ruled out in patients with lower prolactin levels.

Albrecht and Betz noted that out of 352 pregnant patients who had untreated microadenomas, 2.3% had visual disturbances, 4.8% had headaches, and 0.6% had diabetes insipidus. The corresponding figures for 144 pregnant women who had untreated macroadenomas, 15.3% had visual disturbances, 15.3% had headaches, and 1.4% had diabetes insipidus.[12]

Medical treatment for these tumors should be started prior to planning pregnancy.[13] In patients with microprolactinomas, the risk of tumor enlargement during pregnancy is very low, and so these drugs can be stopped as soon as pregnancy is confirmed. However, in patients with macroadenomas, drug withdrawal can result in significant tumor enlargement. These patients require periodic visual field assessment throughout pregnancy.[3] In patients with significant tumor enlargement, medical therapy should be restarted. Surgery should be considered when medical therapy fails.

Bromocriptine can cross the placenta. Krupp and Monka studied data from 2,587 pregnancies in 2,437 women treated during pregnancy with bromocriptine. They did not find an increased risk of spontaneous abortion, multiple pregnancy, or congenital malformation in these patients. In addition, no adverse effect was noted in 988 of their offspring followed-up for 9 years.[14]

Cabergoline is better tolerated than bromocriptine. Cabergoline has been utilized in more than 600 patients in the first trimester, and no adverse effects have been reported.[3]

Breastfeeding stimulates PRL secretion, but there is no evidence that it increases the size of the tumor[3] and, therefore, these patients can continue to breastfeed.[6]

If after 2 years of treatment, serum PRL levels have normalized and magnetic resonance imaging (MRI) shows no tumor, cabergoline can be stopped. These patients, however, require close follow-up.[15]

Cushing's Syndrome and Cushing's Disease

Cushing's syndrome and Cushing's disease are both uncommon during pregnancy. Fertility is usually impaired, because of altered gonadotropin secretion in patients with Cushing's disease and increased adrenal androgen secretion in patients with Cushing's syndrome. Aberrant adrenal LH and hCG receptors probably have a role for the higher incidence of adrenal tumors seen during pregnancy. Recurrent Cushing's syndrome with remission in the postpartum period can also occur.

During pregnancy, approximately 40% of cases of Cushing's due to pituitary adenomas (Cushing's disease), 44% are due to adrenal adenomas, 11% are due to adrenal carcinomas, and the rest are due to pigmented nodular hyperplasia and ectopic ACTH secreting tumors.

The diagnosis of Cushing's syndrome can be difficult during pregnancy because of overlap of symptoms such as edema, weight gain, easy fatigability, hypertension, and impaired glucose tolerance. However the presence of acne, hirsutism, pigmented abdominal striae, easy bruisability, hypokalemia, proximal muscle weakness, and the occurrence of pathological fractures are important clues for the diagnosis of Cushing's syndrome during pregnancy.

Maternal complications include hypertension, diabetes, opportunistic infections, pathological fractures, preeclampsia, premature labor, still birth, and postoperative wound infection. Fetal complications include intrauterine growth retardation (IUGR), prematurity, and suppression of the fetal adrenals.

The loss of normal diurnal rhythm is an important clue for the diagnosis of Cushing's syndrome during pregnancy.[9] Urinary free cortisol levels normally increase up to threefold in the second and third trimester of pregnancy. Urinary free cortisol levels more than 3 times normal indicate underlying Cushing's syndrome. In patients with Cushing's disease, cortisol levels do not respond to low-dose dexamethasone but are readily suppressed with high-dose dexamethasone.

During pregnancy, ACTH cannot be used to distinguish between pituitary and adrenal tumors, as ACTH levels remain normal or high in all forms of Cushing's syndrome, because ACTH is also produced by the placenta. Often these tumors are not identified on MRI scan, inferior petrosal venous sinus sampling (IPSS) has its own limitations during pregnancy.

Medical therapy for Cushing's syndrome during pregnancy is not very effective and is associated with side effects. Ketoconazole is associated with IUGR, metyrapone with hypertension and preeclampsia, aminoglutethamide with fetal masculinization, and mitotane with teratogenicity.

Even though surgery carries a risk for both the mother and the fetus,[9] transsphenoidal surgery or adrenal surgery can be performed in the first trimester of pregnancy. Successful pituitary surgery has also been performed in the second trimester. Early delivery should be considered in the third trimester of pregnancy.

The following features suggest remission of Cushing's disease after transsphenoidal pituitary surgery:[16,17]

- Postoperative cortisol less than 5 μg/dL
- A period of glucocorticoid dependence for more than 6 months
- No cortisol response to CRH or desmopressin [1-deamino-8-D-arginine vasopressin (DDAVP)]
- Restoration of the circadian rhythm and response to dexamethasone.

When transsphenoidal surgery fails, other treatment options include pituitary radiation and bilateral adrenalectomy.[18] Bilateral adrenalectomy can lead to Nelson's syndrome (hyperpigmentation with an expanding intrasellar mass). In a series of 10 patients who had Nelson's syndrome during pregnancy, 5 required postpartum treatment of their pituitary tumor and only 1 required pituitary surgery during pregnancy.[6]

Patients successfully treated for Cushing's disease require lifelong follow-up due to a high incidence of relapse.[19,20]

Nonfunctioning Adenomas

Most of the clinically nonfunctioning pituitary adenomas stain for FSH/LH/α-subunit. During pregnancy, lactotroph hyperplasia contributes to pituitary gland enlargement and this can lead to chiasmal compression in a patient with a preexisting tumor.[3,9]

Hypophysitis

Autoimmune hypophysitis/lymphocytic hypophysitis is commonly associated with pregnancy. Most patients present in the third trimester of pregnancy or in the immediate postpartum period.

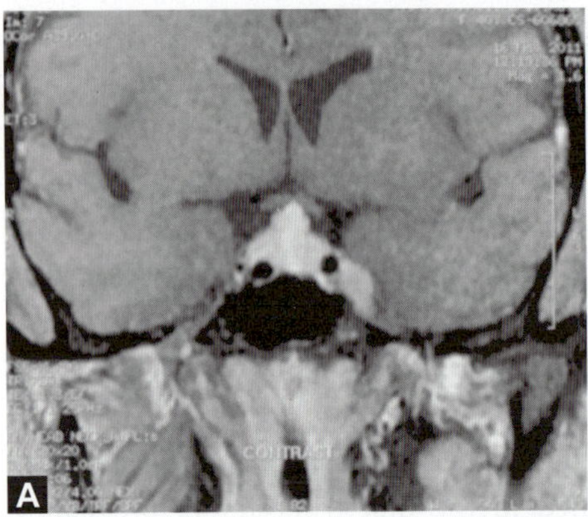

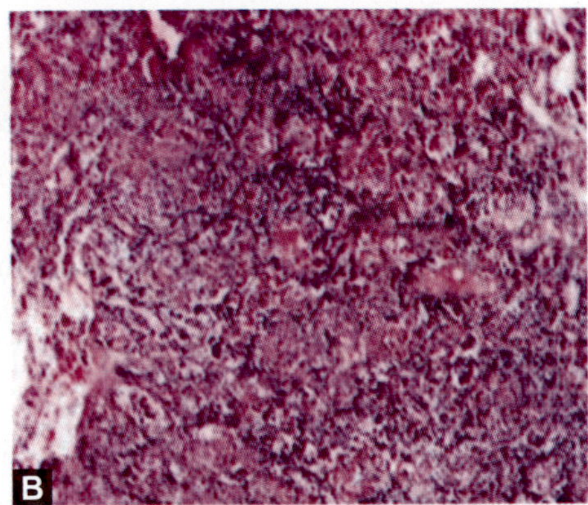

Figure 11-4 Hypophysitis. **A,** MRI appearance. **B,** Lymphocyte infiltration.

Autoimmune hypophysitis is often associated with other autoimmune diseases like Hashimoto's thyroiditis. The symptoms of autoimmune hypophysitis are due to the effects of pituitary gland enlargement and impairment of hormone function. Histopathology reveals mononuclear lymphocytic infiltrates, which progresses to fibrosis (Figure 11-4). Pituitary autoantibodies are detected in up to 70% of these cases.[21,22]

Autoimmune hypophysitis is associated with early destruction of ACTH-producing cells and other anterior pituitary hormones can also be affected; however, posterior pituitary functions are rarely affected.[23]

These patients present with headache and can also have a brightly enhancing sellar mass. They develop hypocortisolism due to early loss of ACTH and rapidly progress to hypopituitarism.[24]

Appropriate management remains controversial. These patients require suitable hormone replacement. High-dose corticosteroid therapy has been tried, which is not very effective. Patients with uncontrolled headache, visual field defects, and progressive tumor enlargement require surgery to debulk the tumor.[21,25]

Hypopituitarism

In patients with preexisting hypopituitarism who are planning for pregnancy, ovulation may be induced with hCG, FSH, and pulsatile gonadotropin-releasing hormone (GnRH).

Hypopituitarism can occur during pregnancy or in the postpartum period, either due to tumor expansion, lymphocytic hypophysitis, or pituitary infarction (Sheehan's syndrome). Pituitary apoplexy is very rare in pregnancy.[26]

Maternal adrenal insufficiency usually does not cause problems with fetal development. On the other hand, fetal cortisol production may protect the mother from severe adrenal insufficiency.

Hypopituitarism can lead to fetal complications like spontaneous abortion and intrauterine fetal death. Maternal complications include hypotension, hypoglycemia, and death in severe cases.[3] Symptoms of adrenal insufficiency may be difficult to recognize, as they are similar to what these patients normally experience in the first trimester of pregnancy—weakness, light headedness, syncope, nausea, and vomiting.

Early morning plasma cortisol levels below 3.0 μg/dL (83 nmol/L) confirms the diagnosis of adrenal insufficiency, and plasma cortisol levels above 19 μg/dL (525 nmol/L) excludes the diagnosis of adrenal insufficiency. Because of high circulating levels of cortisol binding globulin (CBG) in pregnancy, patients with overt adrenal insufficiency may still have plasma cortisol levels in the normal "nonpregnant" range. ACTH levels above 100 pg/mL (22 pmol/L) are found in patients with primary adrenal insufficiency. Because of placental production, ACTH levels may not be suppressed in patients with secondary forms of adrenal insufficiency. The Syanacthen test is not useful in pregnancy.

Glucocorticoid replacement doses are similar to the nonpregnant state. Hydrocortisone is metabolized by 11β-HSD2 in the placenta, and this protects the fetus from overdose. Prednisolone does not cross the placental barrier. In a review of 260 pregnancies in women who received glucocorticoids in pregnancy, two infants had cleft palate.

Patients who are hemodynamically unstable should receive a stat dose of hydrocortisone [100 mg intravenous (IV)] while awaiting the results of confirmatory blood tests. If the diagnosis is confirmed, they should be administered hydrocortisone 50 mg thrice a day, until their clinical condition improves.

Patients who have received long-term steroids are presumed to have HPA axis suppression for 1 year after stopping treatment. They should receive stress doses of hydrocortisone during labor. During lactation, glucocorticoids have the potential to cause growth restriction in the neonate.[6]

Treatment of Hypopituitarism in Pregnancy[5]

Treatment of hypopituitarism in pregnancy is shown in table 11-1.

Sheehan's Syndrome

Sheehan's syndrome results from acute pituitary necrosis following postpartum hemorrhage and shock. Unlike in the past, it is not commonly seen in modern obstetric practice.[27] Pituitary gland enlargement in pregnancy predisposes the gland to ischemia.

Following postpartum hemorrhage, Sheehan's syndrome should be suspected whenever hypotension and tachycardia continue to persist despite adequate replacement of blood products. These women subsequently develop failure of lactation and may experience frequent episodes of hypoglycemia. Postpartum diabetes insipidus can also occur due to involvement of the posterior pituitary gland.[28] Pancytopenia has been reported in rare instances.[29]

TABLE 11-1

Treatment of Hypopituitarism in Pregnancy	
Glucocorticoids	
Maintenance	Hydrocortisone 10 - 5 - 5 mg
	Prednisolone 5 mg morning and 2.5 mg evening
During labor	Hydrocortisone 50 mg IV thrice a day
Cesarean section	Hydrocortisone 100 mg IV before surgery, continue 50 mg IV thrice a day
Thyroxine	
	Eltroxin 0.1–0.2 mg (once daily on an empty stomach)
Vasopressin	
	Tab. Minirin 0.05–0.1 mg twice or thrice daily or
	DDAVP nasal spray 10–20 mg, once or twice daily

DDAVP, 1-deamino-8-D-arginine vasopressin; IV, intravenous.

In milder forms of Sheehan's syndrome, the diagnosis may be delayed for many months or years.[30] These women give a history of failure of lactation, loss of libido, and persisting amenorrhea. They may also complain of fatigue, nausea, vomiting, and diarrhea. Clinical examination reveals breast atrophy, loss of axillary hair, and loss of pubic hair. Some women with partial hypopituitarism have normal menstrual periods and can conceive spontaneously.[31,32]

Investigations to confirm the diagnosis should include ACTH, cortisol, PRL, and free T_4. In the immediate postpartum period, ACTH stimulation test will not be useful, as the adrenal cortex will still respond to stimulation. As T_4 has a long half-life (7 days), its levels may remain normal in the immediate postpartum period. These patients also have low PRL levels. Radiology reveals a partial or empty sella.[3]

These patients should be treated with saline and stress doses of hydrocortisone (50 mg IV 3 times a day). Once stabilized, they are started on oral glucocorticoid replacement. It is important to avoid T_4 prior to starting glucocorticoid replacement, as it can precipitate hypoadrenal crisis in patients with cortisol deficiency.

In a review of 15 pregnancies in patients who had Sheehan's syndrome and had received hormonal therapy, there were 2 (13%) miscarriages and no stillbirths or maternal deaths. In contrast, in 24 pregnancies among 11 women who had Sheehan's syndrome but no hormonal treatment, there were 10 (42%) miscarriages, 1 stillbirth, and 3 maternal deaths.[28]

POSTERIOR PITUITARY DISORDERS

During pregnancy, the set point for a anti-diuretic hormone (ADH) release is reduced by 5–10 mOsm/kg. As a result these women experience thirst and release ADH at much lower levels of plasma osmolality as compared to nonpregnant women

(275 vs. 285 mOsm/kg). This seems to be secondary to high circulating levels of hCG. The placenta also produces vasopressinase, an enzyme, which inactivates ADH and increases the metabolic clearance of this hormone.

Diabetes Insipidus

Patients can present with diabetes insipidus during pregnancy or in the postpartum period.[33,34] Pregnancy can cause exacerbation of preexisting mild or overt diabetes insipidus, which can be due to ADH deficiency (central diabetes insipidus), increased placental degradation by vasopressinase (gestational diabetes insipidus), or ADH resistance (nephrogenic diabetes insipidus).

Central diabetes insipidus may be idiopathic or secondary to a pituitary adenoma, lymphocytic hypophysitis, Langerhans' cell histiocytosis, or sarcoidosis. Patients with idiopathic central diabetes insipidus can have normal fertility. DDAVP, an analogue of ADH, is not degraded by placental vasopressinase and is the drug of choice for treatment.[33] No adverse events have been reported.

Transient diabetes insipidus in the third trimester of pregnancy can occur due to overactivity of placental vasopressinase.[33]

Transient nephrogenic diabetes insipidus in pregnancy has also been reported. Thiazide diuretics are the mainstay of treatment.

Hepatic dysfunction like acute hepatitis, acute fatty liver of pregnancy, and hemolytic anemia, elevated liver enzymes, low platelets (HELLP) syndrome can be associated with transient diabetes insipidus.[34] These symptoms usually resolve by 4th week postpartum.

CONCLUSION

The clinical presentation of pituitary disorders in pregnancy can be very subtle. It is important that these disorders are recognized early. Prompt treatment can prevent maternal and fetal morbidity and mortality.

REFERENCES

1. Karaca Z, Tanriverdi F, Unluhizarci K, Kelestimur F. Pregnancy and pituitary disorders. *Eur J Endocrinol.* 2010;162:453-75.
2. Beckers A, Stevenaert A, Foidart JM, Hennen G, Frankenne F. Placental and pituitary growth hormone secretion during pregnancy in acromegalic women. *J Clin Endocrinol Metab.* 1990;71:725-31.
3. Molitch ME. Pituitary and adrenal disorders of pregnancy. In: Carr BR ed. Endocrinology of pregnancy. Available from: http://www.endotext.org/pregnancy/pregnancy2/pregnancy frame2.htm.

4. Polli N, Pecori Giraldi F, Cavagnini F. Cushing's disease and pregnancy. *Pituitary.* 2004; 7:237-41.
5. Sack J. Thyroid function in pregnancy-maternal-fetal relationship in health and disease. *Pediatr Endocrinol Rev.* 2003;1:170-6.
6. Nader S. Thyroid disease and other endocrine disorders in pregnancy. *Obstet Gynecol Clin North Am.* 2004;31:257-85.
7. Caron P. Acromegaly and pregnancy. *Ann Endocrinol (Paris).* 2011;72:282-6.
8. Bétéa D, Valdes Socin H, Hansen I, Stevenaert A, Beckers A. Acromegaly and pregnancy. *Ann Endocrinol (Paris).* 2002;63:457-63.
9. Molitch ME. Pituitary disorders during pregnancy. *Endocrinol Metab Clin North Am.* 2006;35:99-116.
10. Kars M, Dekkers OM, Pereira AM, Romijn JA. Update in prolactinomas. *Neth J Med.* 2010;68:104-12.
11. Colao A. Pituitary tumors: the prolactinoma. *Best Pract Res Clin Endocrinol Metab.* 2009;23:575-96.
12. Albrecht BH, Betz G. Prolactin secreting pituitary tumors and pregnancy. In: Olefsy JM, Robbins RJ, eds. Contemporary issues in endocrinology and metabolism: prolactinomas. New York: Churchill Livingstone; 1986. p. 195.
13. Ciccarelli E, Camanni F. Diagnosis and drug therapy of prolactinoma. *Drugs.* 1996;51: 954-65.
14. Krupp P, Monka C. Bromocriptine in pregnancy: safety aspects. *Klin Wochenschr.* 1987;65: 823-7.
15. Sedda A, Meyer P. Management of prolactinomas: what's new in 2010? *Rev Med Suisse.* 2011;7:20-4.
16. Czepielewski MA, Rollin GA, Casagrande A, Ferreira NP. Criteria of cure and remission in Cushing's disease: an update. *Arq Bras Endocrinol Metabol.* 2007;51:1362-72.
17. Krikorian A, Abdelmannan D, Selman WR, Arafah BM. Cushing disease: use of perioperative serum cortisol measurements in early determination of success following pituitary surgery. *Neurosurg Focus.* 2007;23:E6.
18. Bertagna X, Guignat L, Groussin L, Bertherat J. Cushing's disease. *Best Pract Res Clin Endocrinol Metab.* 2009;23:607-23.
19. De Martin M, Pecori Giraldi F, Cavagnini F. Cushing's disease. *Pituitary.* 2006;9:279-87.
20. Nieman LK, Ilias I. Evaluation and treatment of Cushing's syndrome. *Am J Med.* 2005;118: 1340-6.
21. Kramp T, Hagen C. Autoimmune hypophysitis. *Ugeskr Laeger.* 2012;172:875-80.
22. Foyouzi N. Lymphocytic adenohypophysitis. *Obstet Gynecol Surv.* 2011;66:109-13.
23. Rivera JA. Lymphocytic hypophysitis: disease spectrum and approach to diagnosis and therapy. *Pituitary.* 2006;9:35-45.
24. Honegger J, Fahlbusch R, Bornemann A, Hensen J, Buchfelder M, Müller M, et al. Lymphocytic and granulomatous hypophysitis: experience with nine cases. *Neurosurgery.* 1997;40:713-22.
25. Molitch ME, Gillam MP. Lymphocytic hypophysitis. *Horm Res.* 2007;68:145-50.
26. de Heide LJ, van Tol KM, Doorenbos B. Pituitary apoplexy presenting during pregnancy. *Neth J Med.* 2004;62:393-6.

27. Kelestimur F. Sheehan's syndrome. *Pituitary*. 2003;6:181-8.
28. Tersnow AH, Wilson JD. The changing face of Sheehan's syndrome. *Am J Med Sci*. 2010; 340:402-6.
29. Laway BA, Bhat JR, Mir SA, Khan RS, Lone MI, Zargar AH. Sheehan's syndrome with pancytopenia-complete recovery after hormone replacement. *Ann Hematol*. 2010;89:305-8.
30. Zargar AH, Wani AI, Laway BA, Masoodi SR, Salahuddin M. Regular ovulatory menstrual cycles in a case of Sheehan's syndrome. *J Assoc Physicians India*. 1998;46:474-5.
31. Zargar AH, Masoodi SR, Laway BA, Sofi FA, Wani AI. Pregnancy in Sheehan's syndrome: a report of three cases. *J Assoc Physicians India*. 1998;46:476-8.
32. Corenblum B. Pituitary Disease and Pregnancy. Available from URL: http://emedicine.medscape.com/article/127650-overview
33. Ananthakrishnan S. Diabetes insipidus in pregnancy: etiology, evaluation and management. *Endocr Pract*. 2009;15:377-82.
34. Aleksandrov N, Audibert F, Bedard MJ, Mahone M, Goffinet F, Kadoch IJ. Gestational diabetes insipidus: a review of an under diagnosed condition. *J Obstet Gynaecol Can*. 2010;32:225-31.

12

Adrenal Disorders in Pregnancy

Sarita Bajaj

INTRODUCTION

Adrenal disorders are relatively uncommon during pregnancy and may be difficult to diagnose because of the alteration of endocrine metabolism and feedback mechanisms of hormones of the mother by the fetoplacental unit. The hypermetabolic state of pregnancy may affect the manifestation of the disease, making it difficult to diagnose. However, timely diagnosis and treatment can prevent significant maternal and fetal morbidity.

ADRENAL FUNCTIONS DURING PREGNANCY

There is a profound effect of pregnancy on adrenal steroidogenesis. The steroid metabolism in the maternal adrenal glands is substantially modified, even though there are no significant morphological changes during pregnancy. In contrast to the hypothalamic-pituitary-adrenal (HPA) axis, a positive feedback is provided by the glucocorticoid levels on the placental corticosteroid axis. Placental corticotropin releasing hormone (CRH) rises hundredfolds during pregnancy resulting in a dramatic rise of both maternal and placental adrenocorticotropic hormone (ACTH) and cortisol levels.[1] The fetoplacental unit has a marked capacity for steroidogenesis, resulting in an increase of plasma cortisol levels (2–3 times the levels of nonpregnant controls) during the course of pregnancy. Plasma 17-hydroxysteroids also increase during pregnancy. A normal maternal circadian rhythm of ACTH persists throughout pregnancy despite the rise in placental hormones and increased HPA axis' function.[2]

Plasma renin activity (PRA) rises early in the first trimester, levels reaching 3–7 times above the normal range by the third trimester. Plasma aldosterone levels increase 5–20 times during gestation. Cortisol rises 2–3 times resulting in a corresponding increase in levels of corticosterone, deoxycortisol, and cortisone. There is a 2 times increase in early pregnancy in the levels of deoxycorticosterone, to 60–100 ng/100 mL in the third trimester, which results in retention of sodium during pregnancy.[3]

CUSHING'S SYNDROME

Cushing's syndrome is extremely infrequent during pregnancy, probably due to hypercortisolism, which inhibits normal ovulation. Gonadotropin secretion is altered in pituitary disease whereas secretion of adrenal androgens occurs in adrenal disease. Approximately, 140 cases of Cushing's syndrome in pregnancy have been reported till date. The incidence of adrenal and pituitary diseases in pregnant women is quite different from nonpregnant women. Out of the total number of cases of Cushing's syndrome, adrenal adenomas comprised almost 40–50% of cases in pregnancy compared with almost 15% of cases in nonpregnant women.[4] Adrenocortical tumors are more frequent in women, with a sex ratio of 4:2. Adrenocortical carcinoma is a rare tumor with an estimated incidence of 1–2 cases/million adults. On the other hand, Cushing's disease comprises over 30% of cases in pregnant women compared with 58–70% in nonpregnant women. It is followed by adrenal carcinoma in about 10% with the rest due to ACTH-independent hyperplasia, ectopic ACTH secretion, and unspecified causes. Recurrence of Cushing's syndrome along with postpartum remission has also been reported.[5]

Symptomatology

As the typical symptomatology of Cushing's syndrome mimics that of pregnancy, it becomes a challenging job to diagnose it during pregnancy. The symptoms include central weight gain, edema, fatigue, emotional distress, hypertension, and glucose intolerance. Hyperpigmented violaceous striae as opposed to skin-colored striae, easy bruising, acne, and hirsutism due to a significant elevation of adrenal androgens are some of the signs and symptoms that help in differentiating Cushing's syndrome from normal pregnancy. Pathologic fractures have also been described.[6]

Diagnosis

Making a biochemical diagnosis of Cushing's syndrome in pregnancy is difficult. The physiologically raised levels of total serum cortisol, serum and urine free cortisol, and ACTH during pregnancy may complicate the diagnosis. In addition to this, the raised levels cannot be suppressed with low doses of dexamethasone (1 mg) but with high doses of dexamethasone (8 mg) during the third trimester.[7] In cases of adrenal adenomas, the levels of plasma cortisol cannot be suppressed even with high doses of dexamethasone. Highly variable responses of ACTH suppression are observed in patients with an ectopic source. In all patients of Cushing's syndrome who are pregnant, ACTH levels have been found to be in the normal to elevated range irrespective of the etiology. This can be postulated due to an increased production of ACTH from placenta and the placental CRH-stimulated production of ACTH from pituitary. Therefore, patients with adrenal adenomas have ACTH levels in the "normal" range, while nonpregnant patients with similar condition have suppressed ACTH levels. Identifying a lack of diurnal variation of free and total cortisol helps in establishing the diagnosis of Cushing's syndrome. In normal pregnancy, even in the presence of elevated cortisol levels, the diurnal variations remain unaltered. Identification of persistently elevated cortisol levels in morning and evening helps in the diagnosis during pregnancy.[8] Radiographic studies are important when there is a biochemical evidence of Cushing's syndrome or Cushing's disease. Pituitary computed tomography (CT) scan or magnetic resonance imaging (MRI) may show more incidentalomas as the pituitary volume usually increases during pregnancy. However, in some cases, a focal abnormality can be identified. The preferred imaging modality for evaluation of the adrenal glands is MRI, as it is safer than CT during pregnancy. Gadolinium, however, is contraindicated.[9]

Complications

The complications of Cushing's syndrome in both the mother and the fetus are severe. These include hypertension, preeclampsia, diabetes, infections, myopathy, muscle wasting, hirsutism, acne, and emotional instability in the mother. Intrauterine growth retardation (IUGR), prematurity, spontaneous abortion, and stillbirths may be seen in the fetus. Premature labor occurs in more than 50% of cases.[7,9]

Female infants have been reported to have masculinization of the genitalia in mothers with adrenocortical carcinoma.

Treatment

Frequency of live births increases from 76 to 89% when treatment is initiated by 20 weeks of gestation. Treatment with metyrapone and ketoconazole is recommended during pregnancy.[7] Surgical therapy is more effective and the preferred form of treatment. Transsphenoidal surgery has been successfully done to treat Cushing's disease. The laparoscopic approach for adrenal surgery has been found to be successful.[10]

ADRENAL INSUFFICIENCY

Adrenal insufficiency is very rare in pregnancy. The most common cause of primary adrenal insufficiency in developed countries is autoimmune adrenalitis, while tuberculosis is more common in the developing world. Polyglandular autoimmune syndrome type 2 [PGA II (primary autoimmune hypoadrenalism or Addison's disease, type 1 diabetes, and thyroid autoimmune disease)] is found more commonly amongst women and more frequent than other forms of PGA. There are several cases of PGA in pregnancy;

with 3 patients presenting with the diagnosis at the time of pregnancy.[11,12] Addison's disease is less common as compared to secondary and tertiary adrenal insufficiency. The most common cause is exogenous corticosteroid administration for asthma, rheumatoid arthritis, etc. The mineralocorticoid deficiency is associated with primary adrenal insufficiency and is not seen in secondary and tertiary disease because the zona glomerulosa continues to be responsive to the actions of renin-angiotensin system.[9]

Symptomatology

The signs and symptoms of adrenal insufficiency like fatigue, dizziness, syncope, nausea and vomiting, weight loss, increased pigmentation, and hyponatremia make the diagnosis difficult, as these are often present in the first trimester of normal pregnancy. Excessive dizziness, syncope, nausea, vomiting, and weight loss should warrant further investigations. Presence of hyperpigmentation on the non-exposed parts of the skin, creases of the hands, the extensor surfaces, and mucous membranes differentiates the hyperpigmentation in Addison's disease from chloasma of pregnancy. Severe salt cravings and decrease in sodium, which is greater than the normal 5 mmol/L decrease in pregnancy, also warrants further evaluation.[13] A study with 5 case reports illustrated that patients presented in stress-induced adrenal crisis in the third trimester, precipitated by illness or labor.[11] An adrenal crisis may usually present in the postpartum period as a result of the protective effect of fetal adrenal production during pregnancy.[12] Careful attention must, therefore, be given to the positive history of autoimmune disorders in the patient and her family members as this would make the diagnosis of Addison's disease more likely.

Diagnosis

Once there is a clinical suspicion, laboratory screening for adrenal insufficiency must be quick. A low early morning cortisol level of less than 3 µg/dL (83 mmol/L) in the non-stressed state and in the setting of a typical clinical presentation is confirmatory. A morning cortisol level of 19 µg/dL (535 nmol/L) in a clinically stable patient in the first trimester and early second trimester excludes the diagnosis.[14] As the normal pregnancy continues, cortisol level rises 2–3 times above nonpregnant level, therefore, a normal morning cortisol level is not common during the second and third trimesters. Hence, patients with a clinical presentation consistent with adrenal insufficiency and a plasma cortisol level of 3–30 µg/dL (83–823 nmol/L) should have further evaluation.[9] When the plasma cortisol level is low for pregnancy and the plasma ACTH level is elevated, primary adrenal insufficiency is diagnosed and synthetic ACTH stimulation testing using Cortrosyn [250 µg intravenously (IV)] should be performed. Adrenal antibodies may be useful in confirming Addison's disease. Maternal adrenal insufficiency causes no problems to the fetus, as the fetoplacental unit has largely autonomous steroidogenesis.

Treatment

Pregnant patients with adrenal insufficiency should be managed using a multidisciplinary approach, including an endocrinologist, an obstetrician, and a pituitary surgeon, if needed. Hydrocortisone is the preferred glucocorticoid replacement treatment, as it does not cross the placenta and only affects the mother. The recommended dose of 12–15 mg/m^2 of body surface area is divided into a twice daily regimen with two-thirds of the dose given in the morning and one-third of the dose given in the afternoon.[15] Routine replacement therapy can be continued until the onset of labor, at which time the oral dose can be doubled. Alternatively, a parenteral dose of 50 mg of hydrocortisone can be given during the second stage of labor, and further dosing can be adjusted based on the progress of labor.[16] Hydrocortisone replacement therapy may be continued during breastfeeding because less than 0.5% of the dose is excreted per liter of milk.[17]

CONGENITAL ADRENAL HYPERPLASIA

Congenital adrenal hyperplasia (CAH) due to steroid 21-hydroxylase (21-OH) deficiency is one of the most common inborn endocrine disorders, accounting for more than 90% of all CAH cases and is inherited as an autosomal recessive disease.[18] Molecular abnormalities of the *CYP21A2* gene coding for the steroid 21-OH enzyme leads to varying degrees of impaired cortisol and aldosterone synthesis and androgen excess. The severity of enzymatic defect is responsible for marked polymorphism of clinical expression. Nonclassical form of CAH (NC-CAH) is due to partial enzymatic defect, and is associated with late onset of symptoms and diagnosis in childhood or after puberty. The classical form of CAH, due to complete or severe 21-OH deficiency, is generally revealed at birth.[19] NC-CAH is much more common than the classical form with an incidence as high as 1:27 in Ashkenazi Jews.[20]

3-β hydroxysteroid dehydrogenase deficiency is the next most common form of CAH, followed by 11-β hydroxylase deficiency, which is followed by the extremely rare forms, 17-α hydroxylase/17, 20 lyase deficiency, congenital lipoid adrenal hyperplasia, and cytochrome 450 oxidoreductase deficiency.[2]

Symptomatology

Females with NC-CAH do not have virilized genitalia at birth; however, many signs and symptoms associated with hyperandrogenemia as seen in classical disease may be seen. NC-CAH is an important and certainly not an uncommon cause of infertility. Adequate glucocorticoid therapy is an important variable with respect to fertility outcomes.

Fecundity and fertility is reduced in women with classic CAH. A summary of various studies on fecundity and fertility in CAH patients is listed in table 12-1.[18,21-28]

TABLE 12-1

Summary of Studies on Fecundity and Fertility in CAH Patients

Study	*No. of patients*	*Age (years)*	*CAH form*	*Summary of key findings*
Mulaikal et al.[21]	80	18–69	SW, SV	Decreased fertility in CAH; adequacy of vaginal reconstruction determines sexual experience
Jaaskelainen et al.[22]	29	16–53	SW, SV	SV females often have irregular menses but final prognosis for fertility overall is good, extremely low child rate in the SW patients
Krona et al.[23]	18	18.3–36.0	SW, SV, NC	Fertility is reduced in females with CAH, especially those with the SW phenotype
Hoepffner et al.[24]	7	22–33	SW, SV	Improvement of pregnancy rate with combination of glucocorticoid and mineralocorticoid replacement
Moran et al.[25]	101	29.7 ± 9.7	NC	Mild subfertility in NC-CAH, increased rate of miscarriages without glucocorticoid replacement in NC-CAH
Hagenfeldt et al.[26]	62	18–63	SW, SV, NC	Pregnancy and delivery rates are reduced in women with CAH mainly due to psychosocial reasons
Casteras et al.[27]	106	18–68	SW, SV	Normal pregnancy rate (91.3%) for women with classical CAH (both in SW and SV); fertility rate lower than in general population
Bidet et al.[18]	190	13–52	NC	Only mild subfertility in NC-CAH; rate of miscarriages is lower in pregnancies occurring with glucocorticoid treatment
Arlt et al.[28]	47	18–69	SW, SV, NC	54% success rate in classic CAH women seeking pregnancy, 67% success rate in NC-CAH women seeking pregnancy

NC, non-classic; CAH, congenital adrenal hyperplasia; HPG axis, hypothalamus-pituitary-gonadal axis; SW, salt wasting; SV, simple virilising.

Childbirth rates are low, but pregnancies are commonly normal and uneventful. CAH results not only in exaggerated levels of 17-hydroxyprogesterone (17-OHP) but also of progesterone, which may interfere with implantation when overtly elevated. Unsatisfactory intercourse due to inadequate vaginal introitus, chronic anovulation due to poorly controlled androgen excess, failure of implantation due to elevated progesterone concentration, and psychological factors, including differences in psychosexual orientation are some of the causes for decreased fertility in women with classic CAH.

Diagnosis and Management

Females with classical disease are aware of their diagnosis before conception and pregnancy. In order to achieve fertility, appropriate control of adrenal hormones with sufficient glucocorticoid therapy is required. In women with NC-CAH, the condition may only be diagnosed during a work-up for infertility, at times after multiple failed *in vitro* fertilization (IVF) cycles. The goal of therapy in CAH is to correct both, the deficiency in cortisol secretion and to suppress ACTH overproduction. The usual requirement of hydrocortisone (or its equivalent) for the treatment of classical 21-OH form of CAH is about 10–15 mg/m^2/day divided into 2 or 3 doses per day with the higher dose given at bedtime. The preferred treatment is hydrocortisone in the affected pregnant female. Nonpregnant women may be treated with the dexamethasone or prednisone, alone or in combination with hydrocortisone. Dosage requirements for patients with NC-CAH are typically less. A small dose of dexamethasone at bedtime (0.25–0.5 mg) is usually appropriate for androgen suppression in NC-CAH patients who are not pregnant; however, as it crosses the placenta, dexamethasone should be avoided in pregnancy. Both prednisone and prednisolone cross the placenta, although in smaller concentrations than dexamethasone. Prednisone is, therefore, less favored in treating nonpregnant patients with CAH.[21] Adequate biochemical control is assessed by measuring serum levels of 17-OHP, androstenedione, and testosterone at a consistent time in relation to medication dosing, usually 2 hours after the morning corticosteroid. Titration of the dose should aim at maintaining androgen levels within the normal range for adult women and 17-OHP levels of less than 1000 ng/dL. Hydrocortisone treatment is suggested during pregnancy when treating the mother with CAH and not the fetus because, unlike dexamethasone, it is metabolized by the placental enzyme 11β-hydroxysteroid dehydrogenase type 2 (11β-HSD2) and does not affect the fetus. 17-OHP and androgens should be assessed at least in every trimester.[29]

Prenatal Management

Administration of glucocorticoids to the mother is used for suppression of fetal adrenal androgens in CAH. Treatment aims to reduce female genital virilization, the need for reconstructive surgery, and the emotional distress associated with the birth of a child with ambiguous genitalia. However, prenatal treatment does not alter the need for lifelong hormonal replacement therapy and the need for careful medical monitoring or the risk of life-threatening salt-losing crises if therapy is discontinued.[30,31]

Fetal cortisol levels are low in early gestation, rise during 8–12 weeks when the external genitalia are differentiating, are only about 10% of maternal levels during mid-gestation, and then, increase during the third trimester. Thus, the constant dexamethasone dose currently used may result in glucocorticoids levels that exceed typical mid-gestation physiological fetal glucocorticoids levels by about 60 times.[32] As CAH is autosomal recessive, if a woman who previously had a child with CAH again becomes pregnant via the same partner, the fetus will have 1 in 4 chances of having CAH. As the period during which the genitalia of a female fetus may become virilized begins as early as 6 weeks after conception, treatment must be started essentially as soon as the woman knows she is pregnant. Dexamethasone is used because it is not inactivated by placental 11β-HSD2. All pregnant women at risk for CAH must start the treatment at 6–7 weeks of gestation. Genetic diagnosis by chorionic villous biopsy cannot be done until 9–11 weeks, even though only 1 in 4 fetuses is affected. Treatment is potentially beneficial for only 1 in 8 fetuses, since only half of the affected fetuses will be females.[33]

Amniocentesis, which is usually performed in the second trimester, may result in a delayed diagnosis as compared to chorionic villous sampling which can be performed at 9–11 weeks of gestation. However, amniocentesis can be used as a reliable alternative method for prenatal diagnosis when chorionic villous sampling is not available.[34]

Treatment is continued till term and discontinued only if the fetus is determined to be a male karyotype or an unaffected female upon DNA analysis. Otherwise, the optimal dosage of dexamethasone is 20 mg/kg/day as per maternal prepregnancy body weight in 3 divided daily doses. It is recommended to start the treatment as soon as pregnancy is confirmed, and not later than 9 weeks after the last menstrual period.[35,36] The mother's blood pressure, weight, glycosuria, glycosylated hemoglobin (HbA1c), symptoms of edema, striae, and other possible adverse effects of dexamethasone treatment should be carefully documented throughout pregnancy. Not only does prenatal treatment effectively minimizes the degree of female genital masculinization in the patients, it also lessens the high-level androgen exposure of the brain during differentiation, which is thought to cause a higher tendency to gender ambiguity in some women with CAH. Genital virilization in female newborns with classical 21-OH deficiency CAH has a potential adverse psychosocial impact that may be alleviated by prenatal treatment.[33]

PHEOCHROMOCYTOMA AND PREGNANCY

High morbidity and mortality in both the mother and the fetus makes pheochromocytoma a rare but important cause of hypertension in pregnancy. Clinically, overt pheochromocytoma during pregnancy may be triggered by several mechanisms. These include increase in intra-abdominal pressure, fetal movement, uterine contraction, process of delivery, an abdominal surgical intervention, and general anesthesia.[37,38] Pregnancy occurs in an age range where vigilance to detect secondary hypertension should always be emphasized.

Diagnosis

All gravidas with chronic hypertension who have not been evaluated for secondary causes should be screened for pheochromocytoma when there is persistence of symptoms and a failure to lower blood pressure despite multidrug maximal therapy. This condition usually mimics preeclampsia (Table 12-2),[39] and maternal mortality can occur when a female with unsuspected pheochromocytoma undergoes an operative delivery. The incidental finding of an adrenal mass along with the "classic" signs and symptoms of pheochromocytoma, i.e., sweating, hyperglycemia, and paroxysmal changes in pulse and pressure should also raise suspicion.[39] Twenty four-hour urinary catecholamines are highly recommended in pregnant patients because pregnancy does not elevate urinary catecholamine levels into the diagnostic range for pheochromocytoma.[40] MRI is the preferred imaging modality because it locates adrenal and extra-adrenal masses and requires no radiation.[41]

TABLE 12-2

Preeclampsia and Pheochromocytoma: Differentiating Features

Features	*Preeclampsia*	*Pheochromocytoma*
Signs and symptoms		
Time of presentation	>20 weeks of gestation	Anytime during pregnancy
Hypertension	Usually sustained	Paroxysmal
Orthostatic hypotension	Absent	Present
Bipedal edema	May be present	Absent
Headache	Usually in more severe preeclampsia	Present
Flushing	Absent	Present
Palpitations	Absent	Present
Weight gain	Present	Absent
Abdominal pain	Present	Absent
Laboratory findings		
Proteinuria	Present	Often absent
Blood glucose	Normal	Increased
Liver transaminases	Elevated	Normal
Catecholamines	Normal	Increased
Thrombocytopenia	May be present	Normal

Adapted from Oliva R, Angelos P, Kaplan E, Bakris G. Pheochromocytoma in Pregnancy: A Case Series and Review. *Hypertension*. 2010;55:600-6.

Management

The primary goal of management is to prevent hypertensive crisis that may lead to both maternal and fetal demise. Medical treatment with α-blocker should be started as soon as the diagnosis is established and should be given for 10–14 days.[42] The drug of choice is phenoxybenzamine, which crosses the placenta and may cause perinatal depression in the mother and transient hypotension in the neonate.[43] Other selective α1 blockers, such as doxazosin, have been used. β-blockers should never be prescribed before α-blockers, as β-blockers alone causes dramatic blood pressure elevations attributed to unopposed adrenergic effects by catecholamines, especially in patients with epinephrine-secreting tumors.[44] Methyldopa is not recommended, as it may worsen the symptoms of pheochromocytoma.[43]

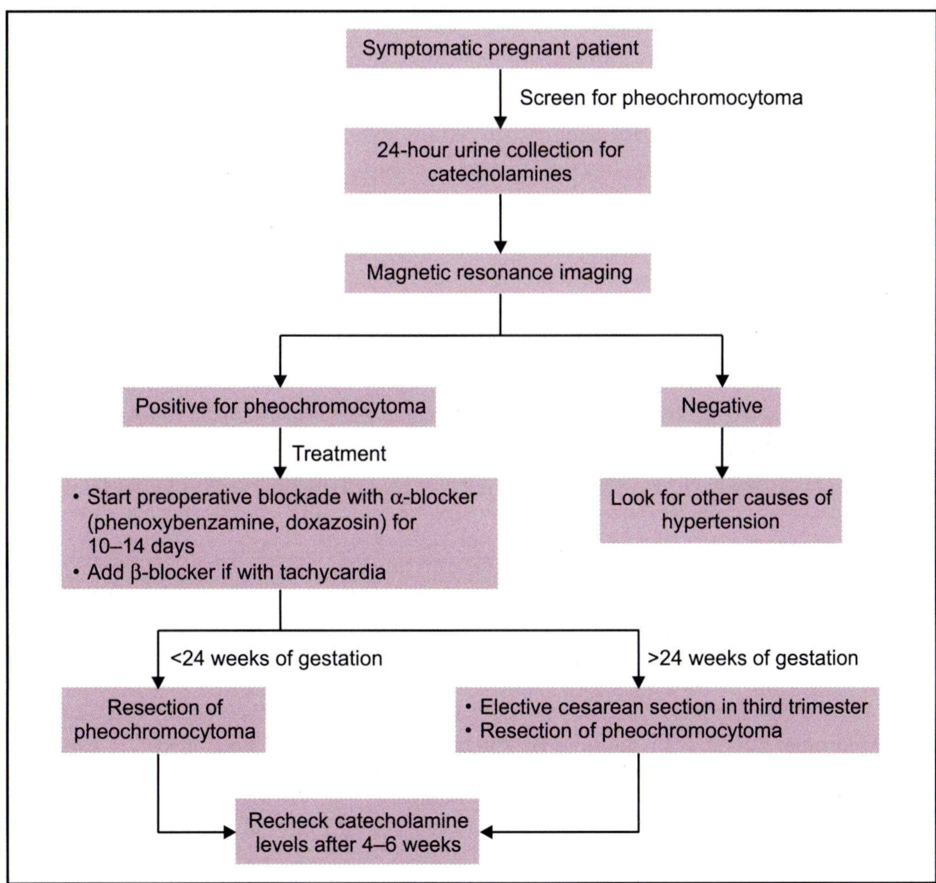

Figure 12-1 Assessment of pheochromocytoma in pregnancy. *Adapted from* Oliva R, Angelos P, Kaplan E, Bakris G. Pheochromocytoma in Pregnancy: A Case Series and Review. *Hypertension*. 2010;55:600-6.

Surgery is the definitive treatment for pheochromocytoma. Gestational age, clinical response to treatment, accessibility of the tumor, and the presence or absence of fetal distress determine the timing of laparoscopic adrenalectomy, which is advocated if tumor mass is less than 7 cm.[43] However, after 24 weeks of gestation, surgical removal is suggested after an elective cesarean section (Figure 12-1).[39] Vaginal delivery carries a higher mortality rate of 31% as compared to cesarean section (19%).[45] The anesthetic approach is also of extreme importance as anesthetic agents can trigger a hypertensive crisis. General anesthesia is safest for the fetus during the second trimester. Early detection and management of pheochromocytoma in pregnancy has resulted in improved fetal outcomes.

CONCLUSION

Adrenal disorders, comparatively infrequent during pregnancy, are a potent cause of maternal and fetal mortality and morbidity, if they remain untreated and undiagnosed. Due to overlapping of the symptoms of adrenal disease with those of pregnancy, it is a great challenge to diagnose them in pregnant women. However, with appropriate investigations, the conditions can be diagnosed early and appropriate treatment can help in saving the lives of mothers and their children.

REFERENCES

1. McLean M, Smith R. Corticotropin-releasing hormone in human pregnancy and parturition. *Trends Endocrinol Metab.* 1999;10:174-8.
2. Lekarev O, New MI. Adrenal disease in pregnancy. *Best Pract Res Clin Endocrinol Metab.* 2011;25:959-73.
3. Dorr HG, Heller A, Versmold HT, Sippell WG, Herrmann M, Bidlinhmaier F, et al. Longitudinal study of progestins, mineralocorticoids, and glucocorticoids throughout human pregnancy. *J Clin Endocrinol Metab.* 1989;68:863-8.
4. Sheeler LR. Cushing's syndrome and pregnancy. *Endocrinol Metab Clin North Am.* 1994; 23:619-27.
5. Buescher MA, McClamrock HD, Adashi EY. Cushing syndrome in pregnancy. *Obstet Gynecol.* 1992;79:130-7.
6. Tajika T, Shinozaki T, Watanabe H, Yangawa T, Takagishi K. Case report of a Cushing's syndrome patient with multiple pathologic fractures during pregnancy. *J Orthop Sci.* 2002;7:498-500.
7. Lindsay JR, Jonklaas J, Oldfield EH, Nieman LK. Cushing's syndrome during pregnancy: personal experience and review of the literature. *J Clin Endocrinol Metab.* 2005;90:3077-83.
8. Aron DC, Raff H, Findling JW. Effectiveness versus efficacy: the limited value in clinical practice of high dose dexamethasone suppression testing in the differential diagnosis of adrenocorticotropin-dependent Cushing's syndrome. *J Clin Endocrinol Metab.* 1997;82: 1780-5.

9. Lindsay JR, Nieman LK. The hypothalamic-pituitary-adrenal axis and pregnancy: challenges in disease detection and treatment. *Endocr Rev.* 2005;26:775-99.
10. Guilhaume B, Sanson ML, Billaud L, Bertagna X, Landat MH, Luton JP. Cushing's syndrome and pregnancy: aetiologies and prognosis in 22 patients. *Eur J Med.* 1992;1:83-9.
11. Albert E, Dalaker K, Jorde R, Berge LN. Addison's disease and pregnancy. *Acta Obstet Gynecol Scand.* 1989;68:185-7.
12. Drucker D, Shumak S, Angel A. Schmidt's syndrome presenting with intrauterine growth retardation and postpartum addisonian crisis. *Am J Obstet Gynecol.* 1984;149:229-30.
13. George LD, Selvaraju R, Reddy K, Stout TV, Premawardhana LD. Vomiting and hyponatraemia in pregnancy. *BJOG.* 2000;107:808-9.
14. McKenna DS, Wittber GM, Nagaraja HN, Samuels P. The effects of repeat doses of antenatal corticosteroids on maternal adrenal function. *Am J Obstet Gynecol.* 2000;183:669-73.
15. van der Spuy ZM, Jacobs HS. Management of endocrine disorders in pregnancy. Part II. Pituitary, ovarian and adrenal disease. *Postgrad Med J.* 1984;60:312-20.
16. Ambrosi B, Barbetta L, Morricone L. Diagnosis and management of Addison's disease during pregnancy. *J Endocrinol Invest.* 2003;26:698-702.
17. Sidhu RK, Hawkins DF. Prescribing in pregnancy. Corticosteroids. *Clin Obstet Gynecol.* 1981;8:383-404.
18. Bidet M, Chantelot CB, Galand-Portier MB, Golmard JL, Tardy V, Morel Y, et al. Fertility in Women with Nonclassical Congenital Adrenal Hyperplasia due to 21-Hydroxylase Deficiency. *J Clin Endocrinol Metab.* 2010;95:1182-90.
19. New MI. Extensive clinical experience: nonclassical 21-hydroxylase deficiency. *J Clin Endocrinol Metab.* 2006;9:4205-14.
20. Speiser PW, Dupont B, Rubinstein P, Piazza A, Kastelan A, New MI. High frequency of nonclassical steroid 21-hydroxylase deficiency. *Am J Hum Genet.* 1985;37:650-67.
21. Mulaikal RM, Migeon CJ, Rock JA. Fertility rates in female patients with congenital adrenal hyperplasia due to 21-hydroxylase deficiency. *N Engl J Med.* 1987;316:178-82.
22. Jaaskelainen J, Hippelainen M, Kiekara O, Vontilainen R. Child rate, pregnancy outcome and ovarian function in females with classical 21-hydroxylase deficiency. *Acta Obstet Gynecol Scand.* 2000;79:687-92.
23. Krona N, Wachter I, Stefanidon M, Roscher AA, Schwarz HP. Mothers with congenital adrenal hyperplasia and their children: outcome of pregnancy, birth and childhood. *Clin Endocrinol (oxf).* 2001;55:523-9.
24. Hoepffner W, Schulze E, Bennek J, Keller E, Willgerodt H. Pregnancies in patients with congenital adrenal hyperplasia with complete impairment of 21-hydroxylase activity. *Fertil Steril.* 2004;81:1314-21.
25. Moran C, Aziz R, Weintrob N, Witchel SF, Rohmer V, Dewailly D, et al. Reproductive outcome of women with 21-hydroxylase-deficient nonclassic adrenal hyperplasia. *J Clin Endocrinol Metab.* 2006;91:3451-6.
26. Hagenfeldt K, Janson PO, Holmdahl G, Falhammar H, Filipsson H, Frisen I, et al. Fertility and pregnancy outcome in women with congenital adrenal hyperplasia due to 21-hydroxylase deficiency. *Hum Reprod.* 2008;23:1607-13.
27. Casteras A, DeSilva P, Rumsby G, Conway GS. Reassessing fecundity in women with classical congenital adrenal hyperplasia (CAH): normal pregnancy rate but reduced fertility rate. *Clin Endocrinol (oxf).* 2009;70:833-7.

28. Arlt W, Willis DS, Wild SH, Krona N, Doherty EJ, Hahner S, et al. Health status of adults with congenital adrenal hyperplasia: a cohort study of 203 patients. *J Clin Endocrinol Metab.* 2010;95:5110-21.
29. Beitins IZ, Bayard F, Ances IG, Kowarski A, Migeon CJ. The transplacental passage of prednisone and prednisolone in pregnancy near term. *J Pediatr.* 1972;81:936-45.
30. David M, Forest MG. Prenatal treatment of congenital adrenal hyperplasia resulting from 21-hydroxylase deficiency. *J Pediatr.* 1984;105:799-803.
31. Forest MG, David M, Morel Y. Prenatal diagnosis and treatment of 21-hydroxylase deficiency. *J Steroid Biochem Mol Biol.* 1993;45:75-82.
32. White PC. Ontogeny of adrenal steroid biosynthesis: why girls will be girls. *J Clin Invest.* 2006;116:872-4.
33. Speiser PW, Azziz R, Baskin LS, Ghizzoni L, Hensle TW, Merke DP, et al. Congenital adrenal hyperplasia due to steroid 21-hydroxylase deficiency: an Endocrine Society clinical practice guideline. *J Clin Endocrinol Metab.* 2010;95:4133-60.
34. Mao R, Nelson L, Kates R, Miller CE, Donaldson DL, Tang W, et al. Prenatal diagnosis of 21-hydroxylase deficiency caused by gene conversion and rearrangements: pitfalls and molecular diagnostic solutions. *Prenat Diagn.* 2002;22:1171-6.
35. Mercado AB, Wilson RC, Cheng KC, Wei JQ, New MI. Prenatal treatment and diagnosis of congenital adrenal hyperplasia owing to steroid 21-hydroxylase deficiency. *J Clin Endocrinol Metab.* 1995;80:2014-20.
36. Carlson AD, Obeid JS, Kanellopoulou N, Wilson RC, New MI. Congenital adrenal hyperplasia: update on prenatal diagnosis and treatment. *J Steroid Biochem Mol Biol.* 1999;69:19-29.
37. Dugas G, Fuller J, Singh S, Watson J. Pheochromocytoma and pregnancy: a case report and review of anesthetic management. *Can J Anaesth.* 2004;51:134-8.
38. Ahlawat SK, Jain S, Kumari S, Varma S, Sharma BK. Pheochromocytoma associated with pregnancy: case report and review of the literature. *Obstet Gynecol Surv.* 1999;54:728-37.
39. Oliva R, Angelos P, Kaplan E, Bakris G. Pheochromocytoma in Pregnancy: a case series and review. *Hypertension.* 2010;55:600-6.
40. Manger WM, Eisenhofer G. Pheochromocytoma: diagnosis and management update. *Curr Hypertens Rep.* 2004;6:477-84.
41. Kennelly MM, Ball SG, Robson V, Blott MJ. Difficult alpha-adrenergic blockade of a phaeochromocytoma in a twin pregnancy. *J Obstet Gynaecol.* 2007;27:729-30.
42. Kinney MA, Narr BJ, Warner MA. Perioperative management of pheochromocytoma. *J Cardiothorac Vasc Anesth.* 2002;16:359-69.
43. Kalra JK, Jain V, Bagga R, Gopalan S, Bhansali AK, Behera A, et al. Pheochromocytoma associated with pregnancy. *J Obstet Gynaecol Res.* 2003;29:305-8.
44. Asensio Martin MJ, Pavon Benito A, Barrena Soles J, Zabaleta Zuniga A, Salvador Bravo M. Anesthesia for surgical removal of a pheochromocytoma during the first trimester of pregnancy. *Rev Esp Anestesiol Reanim.* 2009;56:129-31.
45. Kariya N, Nishi S, Hosono Y, Hamaoka N, Nishikawa K, Asada A. Cesarean section at 28 weeks' gestation with resection of pheochromocytoma: perioperative antihypertensive management. *J Clin Anesth.* 2005;17:296-9.

13

PCOS and Pregnancy

Sarita Bajaj

INTRODUCTION

Polycystic ovarian syndrome (PCOS) is a heterogeneous disorder of unknown etiology, which affects 5–10% of women in the reproductive age group. It is the most common cause of anovulatory infertility and affects the reproductive, endocrine, and metabolic systems.[1] Despite its widespread prevalence, PCOS is a disease with an unclear etiology, varying diagnostic criteria, expansive clinical effects, and debatable management.[2] The first description of PCOS is credited to Stein and Leventhal, who in 1935 made the connection between amenorrhea and polycystic ovaries. In addition, they also noticed the occurrence of masculinizing changes, such as hirsutism and acne, in many patients with polycystic ovaries.[3]

A uniform definition of PCOS does not exist, because of its diverse and heterogeneous nature.[4] In the year 2004, a joint consensus meeting of the American Society for Reproductive Medicine (ASRM) and the European Society of Human Reproduction and Embryology (ESHRE) revised the definition of PCOS. It was agreed that PCOS is primarily a dysfunction of ovary, and, in the absence of other etiologies (such as prolactinoma, congenital adrenal hyperplasia (CAH), or an androgen-secreting tumor), 2 or more of the following criteria establish a diagnosis of PCOS. These criteria are a revision of the Rotterdam criteria (2003) and include:

- Oligo- and/or anovulation
- Clinical and/or biochemical signs of hyperandrogenism
- At least one polycystic ovary on ultrasound.

The morphology of polycystic ovary was redefined as the presence of an ovary with 12 or more follicles measuring 2–9 mm in diameter and/or an increased ovarian volume (>10 cm^3).[1]

EPIDEMIOLOGY

The true prevalence of PCOS is still unknown, because of the preexisting debate about the precise diagnostic criteria. The variations in the data of prevalence are mainly due to inclusion of different populations and diagnostic criteria in the studies. The absence of processes to assess the measures of insulin resistance (IR) in maximum epidemiological studies complicates the situation. The prevalence of appearance of ultrasonic polycystic ovary in hospital-based studies ranges from 45 to 92%. However, community-based studies have reported the incidence of polycystic ovaries to be 17–22%. In a study, it was found that the prevalence of PCOS among the South Asian immigrants in Britain was 52%.[1]

PATHOPHYSIOLOGY

The etiopathogenesis of this syndrome still remains elusive but is likely to be multifactorial consisting of genetic and environmental components.[5] A wide range of theories/systems have been associated in the pathophysiology of PCOS. These include aberrations of the hypothalamo-pituitary-ovarian axis, intraovarian growth factors, fetal programming, and more recently IR and its metabolic consequences, including the metabolic syndrome. A genetic background has also been proposed owing to the increased incidence of symptoms of PCOS amongst family members of the affected women.[1] The evidence in support of the presence of chronic low-grade inflammation in women with this syndrome is emerging. Inflammation is also likely to be associated with other prominent aspects of PCOS, including IR and cardiovascular disease risk factors.[6] IR is the main factor that appears to be quickly gathering pace as a single unifying hypothesis in PCOS.[1] IR is now known to be intrinsic to this disorder, present in approximately 50–70% of the women, independent of obesity, and contributing in a major way to its pathogenesis.[5]

MANIFESTATIONS

PCOS while being clinically heterogeneous, commonly exhibits hyperandrogenism and ovulatory dysfunction and is associated with obesity, IR, and subfertility. Overall, IR and the compensatory hyperinsulinemia affect 65–70% of women with PCOS. In accord with the high prevalence of IR and obesity, glucose intolerance, type 2 diabetes, dyslipidemia, and increased evidence of inflammation are more common in women with PCOS. Similarly, many women demonstrate features consistent with metabolic syndrome and elevated triglycerides, low density lipoproteins (LDL), and decreased high density lipoproteins (HDL) are well recognized.[7]

PCOS AND PREGNANCY

Pregnant women without PCOS have a natural state of IR. With the additive effect of PCOS, the baseline IR may worsen.[2] During early pregnancy, the embryo may be exposed to androgen excess *in utero*. This may have long-term effects, particularly in female offspring. Fetal hyperandrogenism may disturb epigenetic programming, in particular, those genes regulating reproduction and metabolism.[8]

A pregnant woman with a diagnosis of PCOS has several pregnancy-associated complications. These include an increased prevalence of spontaneous miscarriage, gestational diabetes (40–50%) and associated fetal macrosomia, preeclamptic toxemia and pregnancy-induced hypertension (5%), and the birth of small-for-gestational-age (SGA) babies (10–15%).[8,9]

INFERTILITY

The triggering of various metabolic and reproductive abnormalities of PCOS in the affected females is primarily caused by IR. Thecal thickening of ovary is mainly because of elevated insulin levels and associated IR. PCOS may account for more than 75% of the anovulatory infertility.[3] Subfertility in PCOS may be explained by the effects of obesity and/or metabolic, inflammatory, and endocrine abnormalities on ovulatory function, oocyte quality, and endometrial receptivity. Ovarian hyperandrogenism and hyperinsulinemia may promote premature granulosa cell luteinization, and paracrine dysregulation of growth factors may disrupt the intrafollicular environment and impair cytoplasmic and/or nuclear maturation of oocytes. These features are not universal, and oocyte quality, fertilization, and implantation rates in an individual woman with PCOS can be normal.[8] Prevalence of infertility among women with PCOS ranges from approximately 40–75%.[10]

Management of Infertility in PCOS

Multiple approaches have shown to be effective for treatment of infertility in women with PCOS. These include lifestyle modifications, pharmacologic therapy, and surgical interventions.[10] Obesity is observed in 35–60% of women with PCOS and is related to a lack of or delayed response to different treatments, such as clomiphene citrate, gonadotropins, and surgical treatment with diathermy via laparoscopy.[11]

First-line therapy for metabolic dysfunction typically consists of lifestyle modifications including a diet and exercise regimen.[12] Loss of 5–10% of initial body weight in 6 months is sufficient to re-establish ovarian function in more than 50% of obese women with PCOS. Even a less significant amount of weight loss (2–5%) can result in restoration of regular vaginal bleeding consistent with ovulatory patterns.

Short periods (4 weeks) of extremely low-calorie diet (350 kcal/day; 43 g carbohydrates, 33 g proteins, 2.9 g fat per 100 g) can decrease fasting insulin and free testosterone levels and increase the levels of sex hormone-binding globulin (SHBG) and insulin-like growth factor-binding protein type-1 (IGFBP-1).[10]

In selected cases, metabolic surgery in severely obese women may resolve signs and symptoms of PCOS restoring insulin sensitivity and fertility and avoiding long-term risks associated with PCOS and morbid obesity. Before choosing a bariatric procedure, one must consider both the severity of obesity and the possibility of conception in future, since bariatric surgery may help in restoring fertility by sustained and marked weight loss.[13]

Clomiphene citrate is a partially selective estrogen receptor modulator with anti-estrogenic effect in the hypothalamus, where it induces a change in the gonadotropin-releasing hormone (GnRH) pulse frequency. This change results in an increase in follicle stimulating hormone (FSH) level, promoting follicular development and estrogen production. High ovulation rates of 60–85% have been reported with administration of clomiphene and a 30–40% pregnancy rate can be achieved in the first 3 months of treatment.[10] Clomiphene citrate (50–100 mg) taken on days 2–6 of a natural or induced menstrual bleed can be used to induce ovulation. Overall, clomiphene citrate is successful in about 80% of anovulatory women; however, only half of them become pregnant, as these is a reduced effectiveness of clomiphene citrate is obese women with PCOS.[1]

The improved insulin sensitivity and reduction of luteinizing hormone (LH), plasminogen activator inhibitor-1 (PAI-1), and testosterone levels (total and free), which are thought to impair folliculogenesis, have been shown to be achieved by metformin, a biguanide oral antidiabetic drug. FSH and SHBG levels are also increased. The use of metformin is associated with increased menstrual cyclicity, improved ovulation, and a reduction in circulating androgen levels. Metabolic benefits are enhanced in the presence of weight loss, and weight loss itself may be enhanced in the presence of metformin.[11] Metformin can be considered as a first-line agent to induce ovulation in obese and non-obese women with anovulatory infertility caused by PCOS. However, the National Institute for Clinical Excellence (NICE) recommends that in addition to clomiphene, metformin can also be used in women who do not respond to clomiphene alone.[1] Currently, metformin is not recommended as the first-line therapy for infertility in patients with PCOS. The Thessaloniki ESHRE/ARSM Consensus Workshop (2007) advised that, so far, studies do not show an advantage of adding metformin to clomiphene therapy.[10]

Pioglitazone is another insulin-sensitizing drug that has been shown to improve ovulation and increase pregnancy rates. However, fetal safety has not been established [pregnancy category C of the US Food and Drug Administration (FDA) guidelines]. If used, it should be discontinued as soon as pregnancy has been established.[11]

Tamoxifen, another antiestrogenic compound that is very similar in structure to clomiphene citrate, has been evaluated as a fertility agent in the recent past. Ovulation rates have been reported to be 50–90% and pregnancy rates as 30–50%. Tamoxifen has shown reasonably good results in clomiphene citrate failure cases too. The better ovulation and pregnancy rates may be due to higher score of cervical mucus and better functioning of corpus luteum.[14]

As second- and third-line therapies, gonadotropin stimulation and laparoscopic ovarian drilling (LOD) are recommended, respectively for clomiphene citrate-resistant anovulatory PCOS patients.[15] Human recombinant FSH, administered subcutaneously, is frequently used currently. The step-up low-dose FSH induction protocols (37.5–50 IU daily) have shown to be safer for monofollicular development. Due to the recruitment of multiple follicles by gonadotropins, it is found to be allied with an increased incidence of multiple pregnancy and ovarian hyperstimulation syndrome (OHSS). The drawbacks of gonadotropin therapy include its high cost, the need for frequent monitoring of serum estradiol levels, and the need for frequent ultrasound assessments to minimize the risk of development of multiple follicles. The Thessaloniki ESHRE/ASRM Consensus Workshop (2007) recommended a low starting dose of FSH (37.5–50.0 IU daily) with a step-up regimen until 6 ovulatory cycles.[10] Ovarian stimulation has shown to increase the risk of development of perinatal complications.[15]

The pregnancy rates with LOD are low and no case of hyperstimulation of ovary has been reported when compared to gonadotropin therapy. An argument could be made for its consideration before gonadotropins; however, the associated hazards of surgery should be considered. The proposed mechanism of action of ovarian drilling involves a reduction in serum androgen levels due to demolition of the ovarian stroma that produces androgens with electrocautery. This, ultimately, decreases the volume of substrate available for peripheral aromatization to estrogen. It has been postulated that this will restore the feedback mechanism of the hypothalamus-pituitary axis, allowing appropriate gonadotropin stimulation for follicular development and ovulation.[1] Given the invasive nature of these surgical procedures and the development of other medical treatment options, currently these surgical management techniques are seldom used for treatment of infertility.[10]

In patients with PCOS, *in vitro* fertilization (IVF) should be considered in the following indications:

- Failure of nonpharmacologic and clomiphene treatment
- Failure of gonadotropin/intrauterine insemination or
- In cases of a high response to FSH (4 or more follicles) despite low gonadotropin dose.

As in all patients, when PCOS is associated with tubal disease, male factor infertility, severe endometriosis, and/or patients requiring a preimplantation genetic diagnosis, IVF should be considered.[10]

EARLY PREGNANCY LOSS

Early pregnancy loss, defined as miscarriage of a clinically recognized pregnancy during the first trimester, occurs in 30–50% of women with PCOS compared with 10–15% of women without PCOS.[10] The etiology of this association is not known. It may be related to PAI activity, unrecognized hyperglycemia, or a yet to-be-determined factor associated with PCOS itself.[3] Obesity has been conclusively associated with an increased prevalence of miscarriage, and it is obviously more common in PCOS patients than in the normal population. High serum concentrations of LH (>10 IU/L) in the early to mid-follicular phase have been associated with an increased early pregnancy loss in several reports. Clomiphene citrate has a quoted mean miscarriage rate of about 25%. Induction of ovulation with a low-dose FSH protocol also seems to produce a high rate of early pregnancy loss than in the spontaneously conceiving population.[9]

Metformin is capable of reducing insulin concentrations and, consequently, PAI-1 concentrations while not affecting normal glucose levels. In addition, it seems to be capable of enhancing uterine vascularity and blood flow, reducing plasma endothelin-1 levels, increasing luteal-phase serum glycodelin concentration, lowering androgen and LH concentrations, and even inducing weight loss in some patients. These properties would suggest its theoretical clinical utility in the prevention of early pregnancy loss in PCOS, and judging by the results of trials in the last few years, it is becoming a promising treatment option. The evidence so far is that metformin is safe when continued throughout pregnancy, as there has been no increase in congenital abnormalities, teratogenicity, or adverse effects on infant development. The apparent lack of teratogenicity of metformin has earned it an FDA pregnancy category B classification.[9]

Loss of weight by lifestyle changes before pregnancy also improves the rate of early pregnancy loss. GnRH agonists improve the high miscarriage rates. Thus, in addition to weight loss before pregnancy, treatment with metformin has the maximum potential.[9]

GESTATIONAL DIABETES MELLITUS

Considering the high prevalence of obesity and IR among women with PCOS, a higher-than-normal finding of gestational diabetes mellitus (GDM) in PCOS women is expected.[9] IR develops during pregnancy, because of the secretion of human placental lactogen (HPL).[10] The reported reduction in the prevalence of GDM and fetal macrosomia by administering metformin is logical enough to provoke further research into whether this strategy is a feasible option with our present state of knowledge or not.[9]

PREGNANCY-RELATED HYPERTENSION

Pregnancy-induced hypertension (PIH) occurs in 3–5% of pregnancies in previously normotensive women and usually develops during the third trimester. The cause of PIH is likely to be multifactorial, involving immune, genetic, and placental abnormalities.[10] Hypertensive disorders in PCOS may be due to low levels of IGFBP-1 and, therefore, may account for the increase in PIH and preeclampsia.[2] As hypertension is now well established as a possible sequelae of PCOS over the age of 40, especially in those who are obese and insulin-resistant, the trigger of pregnancy is expected to produce an increased incidence of PIH and preeclamptic toxemia (PET).[9]

SMALL-FOR-GESTATIONAL AGE

While the probable association of higher maternal body weight, increased weight gain during pregnancy, and increased prevalence of gestational diabetes in women with PCOS would be expected to produce birth weights higher than the mean, the prevalence of SGA offspring seems to be increased in women with PCOS. IR resulting in impaired insulin-mediated growth and the fetal programming hypothesis are the possible explanations for this higher prevalence of SGA infants in mothers with PCOS.[9]

PERINATAL MORTALITY

Perinatal mortality is increased at least 1.5 times in patients with PCOS.[4]

CONCLUSION

PCOS is a common disorder in women that is associated with significant reproductive and nonreproductive morbidity.[4] PCOS is a complex disease, characterized by variable phenotypes, and whose cause still remains unclear. It is characterized by anovulation, hyperandrogenism, and polycystic ovaries. Infertility is commonly present, and a variety of methods have been used successfully to achieve pregnancy in women with PCOS. Maintenance of pregnancy is complicated by a higher rate of premature spontaneous abortions and an increased risk of GDM, hypertension, and preeclampsia.[10] Immediate diagnosis and preventive therapies are important for the health of women.[4] However, with careful monitoring and treatment, the outcome of pregnancy in most women with PCOS is excellent. Screening of pregnant women with PCOS for GDM, hypertensive disorders, and SGA babies is highly recommended, especially if they are obese, in the light of the increased associations that have been reported.[9]

REFERENCES

1. Bako AU, Morad S, Atiomo WA. Polycystic ovary syndrome: An overview. *Rev Gynecol Pract.* 2005;5:115-22.
2. Kjerulff LE, Sanchez-Ramos L, Duffy D. Pregnancy outcomes in women with polycystic ovary syndrome: a metaanalysis. *Am J Obstet Gynecol.* 2011;204:558.
3. Zisser HC. Polycystic ovary syndrome and pregnancy: is metformin the magic bullet? *Diabetes Spectrum.* 2007;20:85-9.
4. Carmina E, Lobo RA. Polycystic Ovary Syndrome (PCOS): arguably the most common endocrinopathy is associated with significant morbidity in women. *J Clin Endocrinol Metab.* 1999;84:1897-9.
5. Mukherjee S, Maitra A. Molecular and genetic factors contributing to insulin resistance in polycystic ovary syndrome. *Indian J Med Res.* 2010;131:743-60.
6. Duleba AJ, Dokras A. Is PCOS an inflammatory process? *Fertil Steril.* 2012;97:7-12.
7. Marshall JC, Dunaif A. Should all women with PCOS be treated for insulin resistance? *Fertil Steril.* 2012;97:18-22.
8. Fauser BC, Tarlatzis BC, Rebar RW, Legro RS, Balen AH, Lobo R, et al. Consensus on women's health aspects of polycystic ovary syndrome (PCOS): the Amsterdam ESHRE/ ASRM-Sponsored 3rd PCOS Consensus Workshop Group. *Fertil Steril.* 2012;97:28-38.
9. Homburg R. Pregnancy complications in PCOS. *Best Pract Res Clin Endocrinol Metab.* 2006; 20:281-92.
10. Araki T, Elias R, Rosenwaks Z, Poretsky L. Achieving a successful pregnancy in women with polycystic ovary syndrome. *Endocrinol Metab Clin N Am.* 2011;40:865-94.
11. Badawy A, Elnashar A. Treatment options for polycystic ovary syndrome. *Int J Womens Health.* 2011;3:25-35.
12. Duleba AJ. Medical management of metabolic dysfunction in PCOS. *Steroids.* 2012;77: 306-11.
13. Escobar-Morreale HF. Surgical management of metabolic dysfunction in PCOS. *Steroids.* 2012;77:312-6.
14. Dhaliwal LK, Suri V, Gupta KR, Sahdev S. Tamoxifen: An alternative to clomiphene in women with polycystic ovary syndrome. *J Hum Reprod Sci.* 2011;4:76-9.
15. Ott J, Kurz C, Nouri K, Wirth S, Vytiska-Binstorfer E, Huber JC, et al. Pregnancy outcome in women with polycystic ovary syndrome comparing the effects of laparoscopic ovarian drilling and clomiphene citrate stimulation in women pre-treated with metformin: a retrospective study. *Reprod Biol Endocrinol.* 2010;8:45.

14

Obesity and Pregnancy

Sarita Bajaj, Afreen Khan

INTRODUCTION

With increasing prevalence of obesity in both the developed and developing world, more women are entering pregnancy with a high body mass index (BMI) in the overweight (BMI >25 kg/m^2) or obese (BMI >30 kg/m^2) range.[1] The number of inter-related adverse perinatal outcomes in obese women who become pregnant are increasing. Sustained weight retention after pregnancy is an important contributing factor to weight gain among young adult women. A lot of discussion is still going on about the heritability of obesity—the influence of our genetic background vs. environment in the progression of obesity.[2] Now, there is an evidence that the periconceptional period may represent a critical window during which exposure of the oocyte and/or embryo can independently contribute to an increased risk of obesity in the offspring.[1] Several studies have reported that maternal obesity is associated with increased risk for adverse pregnancy outcomes, including gestational diabetes mellitus (GDM), gestational hypertension, preeclampsia, fetal macrosomia, and the need for cesarean delivery.[3] Also, excessive gestational weight gain has been shown to be associated with more postpartum weight retention and development of obesity later in life. Thus, marked obesity is equally hazardous to the pregnant woman and her fetus.

PREVALENCE

The prevalence of overweight and obesity is increasing rapidly among obstetric populations all over the world consistent with broader population trends. Twenty-four percent of women of reproductive age in the UK are now obese and the prevalence appears to be increasing. Studies in these women also show that the rates of obesity in pregnancy have almost doubled in the last two decades.[4] One out of 3 Australian women aged 25–35 years are overweight or obese, 44% of American women in the age group of 18–49 years are overweight or obese, and according to a study, 40% of married women are obese in the United Arab Emirates.[5]

Several clinical and population studies have shown the association between maternal obesity and fertility problems. Suboptimal outcomes for the mother and her fetus during and after pregnancy have been reported with maternal obesity. The association between maternal obesity and an increase in BMI of the fetus in later life, including infancy, childhood, and adulthood has now been proven. The American Heart Association (AHA) Council has recently released a scientific statement in epidemiology and prevention, summarizing the evidence of the prenatal determination of obesity. According to the statement, "*obesity among girls and women of childbearing age is producing a concomitant increase in rates of gestational diabetes, which, in turn, is likely to lead to more obesity in the next generation. This vicious cycle may well fuel the obesity epidemic for decades to come.*"[1]

GESTATIONAL WEIGHT GAIN RECOMMENDATIONS

The Institute of Medicine (IOM) recently released new guidelines for gestational weight gain (Table 14-1) due in part to concerns about the increasing prevalence of obesity in reproductive-age women to better reflect the growing body of evidence in favor of lowering weight gain recommendations for overweight and obese pregnant women.[6] The average weight gain during pregnancy reported in most studies has been 10–15 kg. However, a wide variation is observed in overweight and obese women, in whom many women exceed this average.

The effect of maternal BMI and gestational weight gain has been studied by Cedergren and colleagues[7] in more than 2 lakh women in Sweden. A gestational weight gain of less than 8 kg in obese women was associated with a reduced risk of large for gestational age (LGA) babies, preeclampsia, cesarean section, and operative vaginal birth. However, an increased rate of cesarean section was observed in pregnancies with

TABLE 14-1

Recommendations for Appropriate Gestational Weight Gain Based on Preconception Body Mass Index Given by the Institute of Medicine in 2009

Preconception body mass index (kg/m²)	*Total weight gain (kg) during pregnancy*	*Weight gain (kg) during 2nd and 3rd trimesters (per week)*
<18.5	13–18	0.5–0.6
18.5–24.9	11–16	0.4–0.5
25.0–29.9	7–11	0.2–0.3
≥30.0	5–9	0.2–0.3

Source: Institute of Medicine, Weight Gain during Pregnancy: Reexamining the Guidelines, The National Academies Press, Washington, DC, USA, 2009.

high gestational weight gain in each of the 5 BMI categories. Thus, it was concluded that, as recommended by the IOM, a limited weight gain in pregnancy may be of benefit to obese women. On the other hand, fetal growth and development may be hampered, if there is severe restriction of maternal diet.

Although Cedergren and colleagues have shown that women with less than 8 kg weight gain in pregnancy have a reduced risk of LGA infants, this possibly occurs at the expense of a rise in the number of small for age (SGA) infants with excessively restricted weight gain. Thus, recommendations have been made to avoid weight loss during pregnancy as well as to limit restriction of weight gain to approximately 5 kg throughout pregnancy in obese women.[8]

OBESITY-RELATED OBSTETRICAL COMPLICATIONS

There is an increased risk of complications associated independently with both prepregnancy overweight or obesity and excessive pregnancy weight gain. The association between increased maternal BMI and the high risk of obstetric and neonatal complications has been demonstrated by several studies till date. The whole duration of the peripregnancy period, including antepartum, intrapartum, intraoperative, postoperative, and postpartum period in overweight and obese women, has been shown to be associated with an increased risk of complications.[6]

Maternal Morbidity

Obesity results in increased maternal morbidity. A number of studies[5,9-13] have shown an association between increasing maternal BMI and an increased risk of hypertensive disorders of pregnancy, GDM, induction of labor, cesarean section, longer length of maternal stay in hospital, and increased birth weight (Table 14-2).

Athukorala et al.[10] reported that obese women were at a higher risk of developing preeclampsia, received more magnesium sulfate and antihypertensives, were at higher risk of developing GDM, were more likely to be induced and undergo a cesarean section overall, have an emergency cesarean section, and were more likely to require antibiotics postpartum, when compared to women with normal BMI. It was estimated that every 1 unit increase in BMI among nulliparous women conferred a 7% increase in risk for preeclampsia and a 6% increase in risk for early preeclampsia.[10]

A prospective study by the Atlantic Diabetes in Pregnancy (ATLANTIC DIP) observed that cesarean deliveries increased in overweight [odds ratio (OR) 1.57, 95% confidence interval (CI) 1.24–1.98] and obese (OR 2.65, 95% CI 2.03–3.46) women. Hypertensive disorders increased in overweight (OR 2.30, 95% CI 1.55–3.40) and obese (OR 3.29, 95% CI 2.14–5.05) women. Reported miscarriages increased in obese (OR 1.4, 95% CI 1.11–1.77) women. Thus, overweight and obese glucose-tolerant women had greater incidence of adverse pregnancy outcomes.[11]

TABLE 14-2

Prevalence and Odds Ratios for Pregnancy and Birth Complications				
Pregnancy and birth complications	*Prevalence in normal weight women*	*Prevalence in obese women*	*Range of odds ratios-obese women*	*Range of odds ratios-class II and or III obesity*
Gestational diabetes	1.2–4.1% 14, 17, 18, 54	3.5–9.5% 14, 15, 17, 18, 23, 54	2.6–5.2 15, 16, 18, 20, 23, 54	4–7.4 14, 17, 18
Hypertensive disorders of pregnancy	0.7–4.8% 14, 17, 18	1.4–13.5% 14, 15, 17, 18	2.1–5.2 13, 14–16, 18, 20	3.2–4.9 10, 14, 17, 18
Cesarean section	7.7–22.3% 10, 14, 17	10.4–36.2% 14, 15, 17	1.7–2.9 15, 16, 17, 20	2.5–3.0 14, 16, 17
Premature birth <37 weeks	5.4–19.6% 14, 16, 17, 18	6.4–30.7% 12, 14, 15, 17, 18	0.9–1.6 15, 18, 20, 38	1.5–1.85 17, 18
Special care nursery admission	4.3–9.3% 17	6–33.2% 17	1.2–1.3 16	1.4–3.4 16
Congenital abnormality	1.2–4.5% 16, 22, 23, 36	2.2–5.5% 22–24, 29, 31–33, 36	1.1–2.6 22–24, 36	1.4–3.4 14, 22, 29

Adapted from Nitert MD, Foxcroft KF, Lust K, Fagermo N, Lawlor DA, O'Callaghan M, et al. Overweight and obesity knowledge prior to pregnancy: a survey study. *BMC Pregnancy and Childbirth.* 2011;11:96.

Mamun et al.[5] observed that for each 100 g increase in gestational weight gain, maternal stay in the hospital increased by 0.09 days, i.e., mothers stayed 2.2 hours longer in the hospital, which is equivalent to 1 day longer stay in hospital for every 1 kg increase in gestational weight gain.

However, obesity has been associated with reduced risk for placental abruption when the weight gain during pregnancy is moderate.[14]

Long-term Consequences in Mother

Excessive prepregnancy weight can be used to predict long-term obesity with its attendant morbidity and mortality. Rooney and Schanberger[15] reported that excess weight gain during pregnancy, and not prepregnancy weight, is a predictor of long-term obesity.[15]

Perinatal Morbidity

The complications in the neonates associated with maternal obesity include macrosomia (birth weight >4 kg), fetal distress, shoulder dystocia, and perinatal morbidity or mortality. Stillbirth and birth defects, such as cleft palate, omphalocele, hydrocephaly, and heart and neural tube defects are the disastrous neonatal outcomes ascribed to maternal obesity. Detection of anomalies is even more difficult, because of the technical challenges of ultrasound in obese women.

Macrosomic neonates born to obese mothers are at an increased risk of birth injury, hyaline membrane disease, meconium aspiration syndrome, and require more assisted ventilation.[6] An increase in the prepregnancy BMI between two successive pregnancies results in an overall elevated risk of stillbirth, with the highest risk of stillbirth seen among women with a BMI that changed from normal to obese between two consecutive pregnancies.[16] Prepregnancy maternal obesity has also been associated with increased risk of infant death.[17] The offsprings of obese women have been shown to have significantly higher OR for atrial septal defects, hypoplastic left heart syndrome, aortic stenosis, pulmonic stenosis, and tetralogy of Fallot.[18]

Modifiable intrauterine exposures that influence infant size and rapid infant weight gain, a measure of infant growth rate within the first 6 months of life, are prepregnancy BMI and gestational weight gain. Infants of overweight and obese mothers have more weight relative to their length.[19]

The risks of preterm birth and induced preterm birth is increased in overweight and obese women with an overall increased risk of preterm birth.[20]

Long-term Consequences in Child

Maternal environment, especially during early fetal life seems to have a determinant role in the tendency to develop various abnormalities in the offspring (Figure 14-1).

Maternal body weight, overnutrition, or a high fat consumption during pregnancy is associated with the development of components of the metabolic syndrome, cardiovascular and renal disease, hypertension, and cerebral dysfunction as well as type 2 diabetes and obesity themselves later in the life of the progeny.[21] Moreover, offspring from obese women are more likely to develop obesity, diabetes mellitus, and cardiovascular diseases at a younger age in their lifetime.[22]

Fetal programming of metabolic functions, induced by obesity and GDM, may have intergenerational effect and, thus, perpetuate the burden of such conditions. It is usually believed that increased food consumption and changes in lifestyle are responsible for the growing incidence of obesity in our society; however, there is an increasing evidence on the influence of prenatal events influencing the development of obesity during infancy and adulthood. Maternal environment, especially during early fetal life, is also associated with the risk of development of obesity in the offspring (Figure 14-2). The impact of maternal obesity seems to start in the reproductive tissues of the mother: the ovaries show increased apoptotic follicles, smaller oocyte size and number, and delayed meiotic maturation. The preimplantation events are also altered: insulin-like

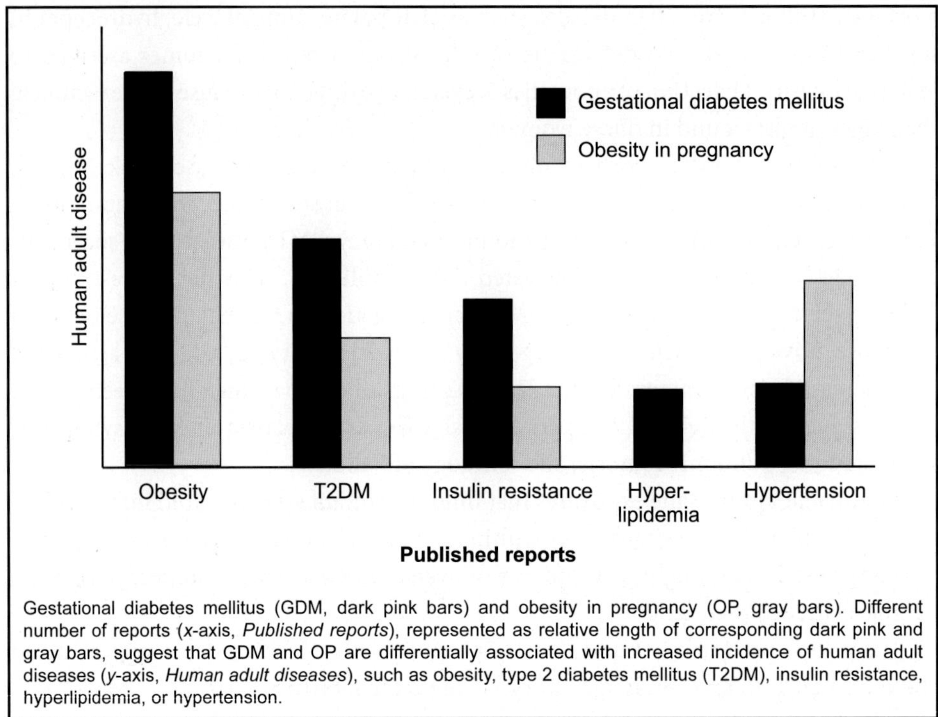

Figure 14-1 Comparison of published reports addressing a potential association of human adult diseases in subjects from pregnancies coursing with gestational diabetes mellitus or obesity in pregnancy. *Adapted from* Leiva A, Pardo F, Ramirez M, Farias M, Casanello P, Sobrevia L. Fetoplacental Vascular Endothelial Dysfunction as an Early Phenomenon in the Programming of Human Adult Diseases in Subjects Born from Gestational Diabetes Mellitus or Obesity in Pregnancy. *Experimental Diabetes Research*. 2011;2011:349286; *with permission*.

growth factor 1 receptor (IGF1R) expression, which is critical for insulin signaling and glucose transport, is blunted in the blastocysts. This correlates to increased apoptosis.[23] Males are more affected than females. At birth, the offsprings of obese women present with higher percentage of body fat, higher insulin resistance (IR), and higher leptin and interleukin (IL)-6, suggesting that maternal obesity results in a higher risk for the progeny with metabolic insults already at birth.[24]

Overweight or obese women give birth to macrosomic girls, who are more likely to become obese themselves and deliver large-sized neonates. Thus, prepregnancy obesity and excessive gestational weight gain results in an intergenerational "vicious cycle" of obesity. Children of obese women exhibit increased risk of diabetes in pregnancy, increasing the likelihood of development of IR in later life.[25]

A number of studies have linked obesity with asthma in adults and children. Children of obese mothers have shown to have an increased risk of recurrent wheezing.[26]

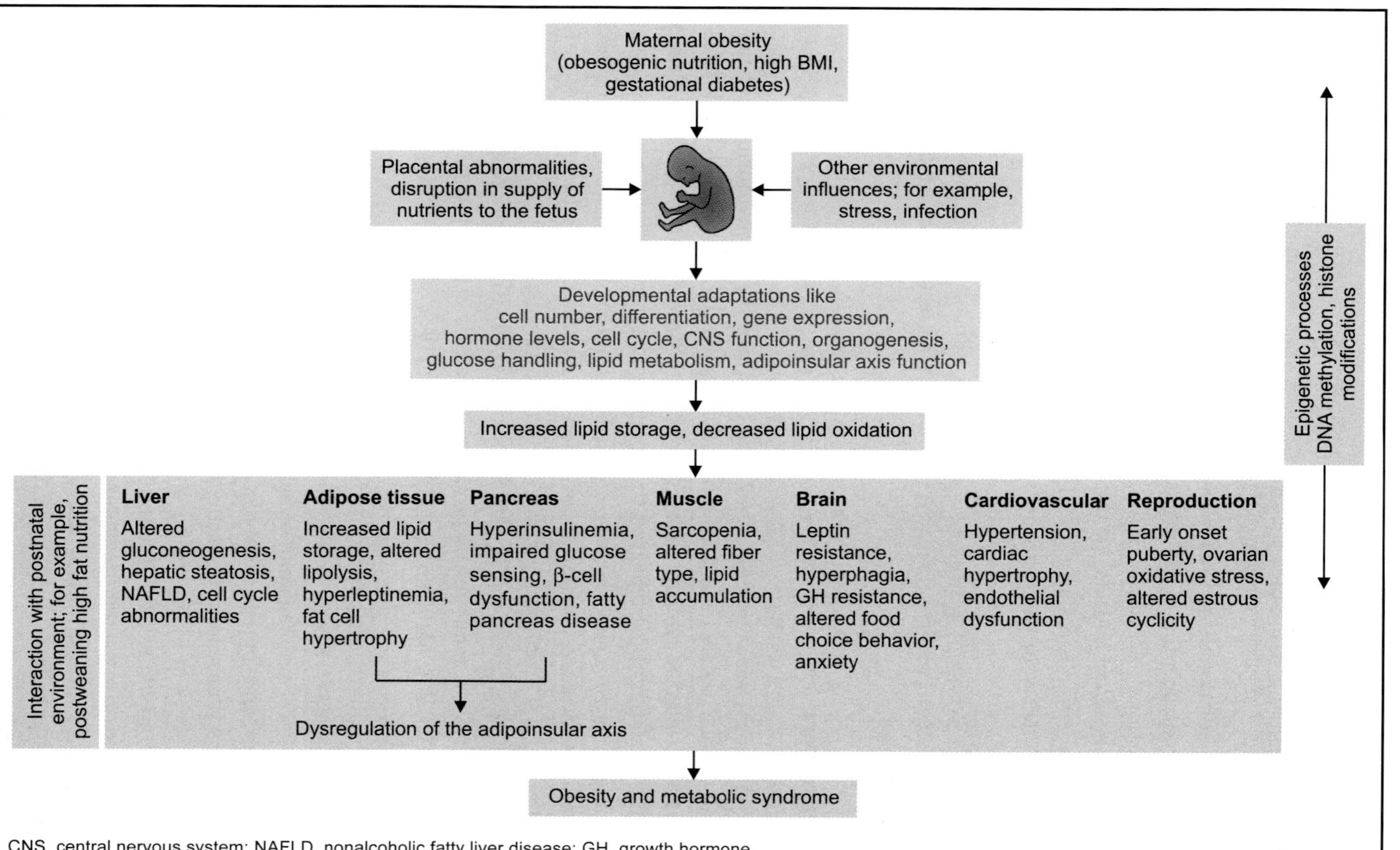

CNS, central nervous system; NAFLD, nonalcoholic fatty liver disease; GH, growth hormone.

Figure 14-2 A schematic presentation of consequences of a maternal obesogenic environment on the health and well-being of offspring.

CONTRACEPTION AND OBESITY

Unplanned pregnancy is of greater concern in a population at high risk for complications during pregnancy. In addition, counseling for contraceptive options in obese women seems to be more complex than in women with normal weight. The combined hormonal methods may have a higher failure rate in obese women. Intrauterine contraception device placement as well as surgical sterilization is more challenging technically, and both have greater chances of resulting in complications in obese women, in spite of high contraceptive efficacy. The risk of venous thromboembolism is elevated in obese women who use combined hormonal contraception relative to women who are not using them, though the absolute risk is small.

Additionally, achieving pregnancy can be more difficult for obese women because they are less likely to ovulate regularly, have decreased fecundity, and have increased risk of miscarriage.[27]

MANAGEMENT

Since most women are concerned about the health of their baby during pregnancy and are in regular contact with their healthcare providers during this period, it is an opportune period to educate them in order to promote healthy diet and physical activity. Research has also established the benefits of healthy diet and physical activity during pregnancy to gain the recommended amount of weight during pregnancy, which would help make a major contribution in preventing weight retention in the postpartum period. According to observational data, interpregnancy weight loss is associated with a decreased risk of preeclampsia, LGA infants, and cesarean delivery.[2] A program of weight reduction is probably unrealistic during pregnancy. If such a regimen is chosen, it is mandatory that the quality of the diet be monitored closely and ketosis be avoided.

Currently, 30 minutes of physical activity is recommended on most days of the week to all pregnant women having no medical or obstetric complications. Obese pregnant women with a lower prepregnancy weight, a history of spontaneous abortion, having children at home, and those without nausea, vomiting, or low backache, are most likely to be advised to exercise in early pregnancy.[28]

Most early signs of hypertension or diabetes may be detected by close prenatal surveillance. Serial sonography is required for the accurate assessment of fetal growth. It is mandatory to give the required attention to complications that might occur during labor and delivery. Preplanning with regard to the type and placement of abdominal incision to access the fetus and the intervening tissue thickness is necessary in case of cesarean delivery.

SCREENING FOR OBESITY

Obesity is considered to be a disease with significant impact on public health in the reproductive years as well as in the later life. In spite of this fact, screening for obesity in general and in women of reproductive age in particular remains an understudied intervention. There are enough data available now, which support the basic criteria for screening for obesity in women in the reproductive age group. Calculation of BMI for screening for obesity is a simple, cheap, and easily reproducible technique that estimates adiposity reliably. The theoretical risks of stigma associated with diagnosis, misdiagnosis, and treatment cost have not yet been demonstrated in available literature.

Appropriate treatment with resultant weight loss is a potential advantage of screening, which may improve outcomes for women and their children. Weight loss occurring before pregnancy, even if it is not sustained over time, is associated with reduced maternal morbidity and decreased role of long-term cardiometabolic consequences in children. Therefore, at least appropriate preconception counseling is possible, if obesity is identified before contraception. The American Congress of Obstetricians and Gynecologists (ACOG) recommends counseling regarding the benefits of weight reduction, discussion of maternal and fetal risks of obesity in prepregnancy period, and appropriate management to identify early and minimize possible complications of obesity.[27]

CONCLUSION

The intrauterine environment and nutritional conditions during fetal life may be considered as epigenetic mechanisms that could play a role in the development of obesity during adult life.[29] The epigenetic modifications alter gene functions (silencing or activating) without changes in DNA. These are caused by environmental agents, including nutrition, pollutants, and other agents and are heritable. Further research is needed on the specific events that take place in obesity during pregnancy, such as DNA methylation or histone acetylation. One of the best candidates for epigenetic modifications in diabetes and obesity is nutrition.[30] This means that not only genetic factors or familial environment contribute to the development of obesity in the progeny, but also the uterine environment seems to determine the degree of obesity in the progeny born from obese mothers. The uterine environment seems even more important than genetic factors.[31] The efficacy of weight loss interventions in periconceptional period has now been conclusively demonstrated in reversing the impact of maternal obesity on the child. These interventions have a great value in preventing future cardiometabolic risks in the offspring and breaking the vicious cycle of intergenerational propagation of obesity. However, careful consideration with regard to the nature and the timing of intervention is mandatory, since it can by itself induce organ reprogramming and have potential long-term effects on the offspring. Long-lasting metabolic effects on the offspring are seen with reduction of maternal gestational weight gain, even if fetal and neonatal profiles are similar or slightly changed. Thus, it may be concluded that beneficial effects of interventions in humans in the intrauterine environment may have long-lasting effect on health of the offspring in later life even if they may not result in improved newborn phenotype.[6]

It is well established that obese patients who receive healthcare provider's advice about weight loss or strategies for improving diet and exercise are more likely to work on these areas even in pregnancy. There is also a need for more education regarding BMI definitions and weight gain guidelines, along with strategies to address provider-personal factors, such as confidence and body satisfaction that are important predictors of adherence to management recommendations.[32]

REFERENCES

1. Zhang S, Rattanatray L, Morrison JL, Nicholas LM, Lie S, McMillen IC. Maternal obesity and the early origins of childhood obesity: weighing up the benefits and costs of maternal weight loss in the periconceptional period for the offspring. *Exp Diabetes Res.* 2011; 2011:585749.
2. Phelan S. Pregnancy: A "teachable moment" for weight control and obesity prevention. *Am J Obstet Gynecol.* 2010;202:135.
3. Kongubol A, Phupong V. Prepregnancy obesity and the risk of gestational diabetes mellitus. *BMC Pregnancy Childbirth.* 2011;11:59.
4. Oteng-Ntim E, Varma R, Croker H, Poston L, Doyle P. Lifestyle interventions for overweight and obese pregnant women to improve pregnancy outcome: systematic review and meta-analysis. *BMC Med.* 2012;10:47.
5. Mamun AA, Callaway LK, O'Callaghan MJ, Williams GM, Najman JM, Alati R, et al. Associations of maternal pre-pregnancy obesity and excess pregnancy weight gains with adverse pregnancy outcomes and length of hospital stay. *BMC Pregnancy Childbirth.* 2011;11:62.
6. Battista MC, Hivert MF, Duval K, Baillargeon JP. Intergenerational cycle of obesity and diabetes: how can we reduce the burdens of these conditions on the health of future generations? *Exp Diabetes Res.* 2011;2011:596060.
7. Cedergren M. Effects of gestational weight gain and body mass index on obstetric outcomes in Sweden. *Int J Gynaecol Obstet.* 2006;93:269-74.
8. Dodd JM, Turnbull DA, McPhee AJ, Wittert G, Crowther CA, Robinson JS. Limiting weight gain in overweight and obese women during pregnancy to improve health outcomes: the LIMIT randomised controlled trial. *BMC Pregnancy Childbirth.* 2011; 11:79.
9. Yazdani S, Yosofniyapasha Y, Nasab BH, Mojaveri MH and Bouzari Z. Effect of maternal body mass index on pregnancy outcome and newborn weight. *BMC Res Notes.* 2012;5:34.
10. Athukorala C, Rumbold AR, Willson KJ, Crowther CA. The risk of adverse pregnancy outcomes in women who are overweight or obese. *BMC Pregnancy Childbirth.* 2010;10:56.

11. Owens LA, O'Sullivan EP, Kirwan B, Avalos G, Gaffney G, Dunne F; ATLANTIC DIP Collaborators. ATLANTIC DIP: The impact of obesity on pregnancy outcome in glucose-tolerant women. *Diabetes Care.* 2010;33:577-9.
12. Magriples U, Kershaw TS, Rising SS, Westdahl C, Ickovics JR. The effects of obesity and weight gain in young women on obstetric outcomes. *Am J Perinatol.* 2009;26:365-71.
13. Addo VN. Body mass index, weight gain during pregnancy and obstetric outcomes. *Ghana Med J.* 2010;44:64-9.
14. Salihu HM, Lynch O, Alio AP, Kornosky JP, Clayton HB, Mbah AK. Extreme obesity and risk of placental abruption. *Hum Reprod.* 2009;24:438-44.
15. Rooney BL, Schauberger CW. Excess pregnancy weight gain and long-term obesity: one decade later. *Obstet Gynecol.* 2002;100:245-52.
16. Whiteman VE, Crisan L, McIntosh C, Alio AP, Duan J, Marty PJ, et al. Interpregnancy Body Mass Index Changes and Risk of Stillbirth. *Gynecol Obstet Invest.* 2011;72:192-5.
17. Thompson DR, Clark CL, Wood B, Zeni MB. Maternal obesity and risk of infant death based on Florida birth records for 2004. *Public Health Rep.* 2008;123:487-93.
18. Mills JL, Troendle J, Conley MR, Carter T, Druschel CM. Maternal obesity and congenital heart defects: a population-based study. *Am J Clin Nutr.* 2010;91:1543-9.
19. Deierlein AL, Siega-Riz AM, Adair LS, Herring AH. Effects of prepregnancy body mass index and gestational weight gain on infant anthropometric outcomes. *J Pediatr.* 2011;158: 221-6.
20. McDonald SD, Han Z, Mulla S, Beyene J; Knowledge Synthesis Group. Overweight and obesity in mothers and risk of preterm birth and low birth weight infants: systematic review and meta-analyses. *BMJ.* 2010;341:c3428.
21. Maric-Bilkan C, Symonds M, Ozanne S, Alexander BT. Impact of maternal obesity and diabetes on long-term health of the offspring. *Exp Diabetes Res.* 2011;2011:163438.
22. Huda SS, Brodie LE, and Sattar N. Obesity in pregnancy: prevalence and metabolic consequences. *Semin Fetal Neonatal Med.* 2010;15:70-6.
23. Chi MM, Schlein AL, Moley KH. High insulin-like growth factor 1 (IGF-1) and insulin concentrations trigger apoptosis in the mouse blastocyst via down-regulation of the IGF-1 receptor. *Endocrinology.* 2000;141:4784-92.
24. Catalano PM, Presley L, Minium J, Hauguel-de Mouzon S. Fetuses of obese mothers develop insulin resistance in utero. *Diabetes Care.* 2009;32:1076-80.
25. Leiva A, Pardo F, Ramirez M, Farias M, Casanello P, Sobrevia L. Fetoplacental vascular endothelial dysfunction as an early phenomenon in the programming of human adult diseases in subjects born from gestational diabetes mellitus or obesity in pregnancy. *Exp Diabetes Res.* 2011;2011:349286.
26. Kumar R, Story RE, Pongracic JA, Hong X, Arguelles L, Wang G, et al. Maternal pre-pregnancy obesity and recurrent wheezing in early childhood. *Pediatr Allergy Immunol Pulmonol.* 2010;23:183-90.
27. Zera C, McGirr S, Oken E. Screening for obesity in reproductive-aged women. *Prev Chronic Dis.* 2011;8:A125.
28. Foxcroft KF, Rowlands IJ, Byrne NM, McIntyre HD, Callaway LK; BAMBINO group. Exercise in obese pregnant women: The role of social factors, lifestyle and pregnancy symptoms. *BMC Pregnancy Childbirth.* 2011;11:4.

29. Yajnik CS, Godbole K, Otiv SR, Lubree HG. Fetal programming of type 2 diabetes: Is sex important? *Diabetes Care*. 2007;30:2754-5.
30. McCurdy CE, Bishop JM, Williams SM, Grayson BE, Smith MS, Friedman JE, et al. Maternal high-fat diet triggers lipotoxicity in the fetal livers of nonhuman primates. *J Clin Invest*. 2009;119:323-35.
31. Obregon MJ. Maternal Obesity Results in Offspring Prone to Metabolic Syndrome. *Endocrinology*. 2010;151:3475-6.
32. Herring SJ, Platek DN, Elliott P, Riley LE, Stuebe AM, Oken E. Addressing obesity in pregnancy: what do obstetric providers recommend? *J Womens Health (Larchmt)*. 2010; 19:65-70.

15

Fetal Origins of Endocrine Disease

Senthil Vasan K, Veena Nair, Nihal Thomas

INTRODUCTION

The role of early life events in the genesis of adult diseases has been a subject of great interest in recent years. There is a considerable evidence favoring an inverse association of early life events like birth size and subsequent disease and mortality in adulthood.

Although epidemiological evidence is robust, the underlying mechanisms still remain unclear, and the proposed theories overlap each other. Events that lead to the manipulation of environment extending from conception to infancy appear to be crucial, since these changes lead to permanent structural and physiological alterations leading to a susceptible adult phenotype that is prone to disease.

In the recent past, molecular mechanisms associated with permanent alterations in gene expression and regulated by epigenetic factors have gained considerable importance in recent years. Therefore, understanding the role of early life events, postnatal environmental exposure, and genetic mechanisms would offer new avenues to diagnosis, prevention, and management of adult disease. In the current chapter, we will discuss clinical and experimental evidence that favor early life events and adult diseases with particular relevance to endocrine disorders.

DEVELOPMENTAL ORIGINS OF HEALTH AND DISEASE

The "developmental origins of health and disease" (DOHaD) paradigm emphasizes that certain factors (nutrition, environment) have a developmental impact during the critical period of early life, and these influence adult disease outcomes.[1,2] The earliest evidence of DOHaD appears from the epidemiological observations by Barker et al. (1986)[1] and Hales et al. (1991)[2] relating birth size and risk of cardiovascular disease and type 2 diabetes, respectively in adulthood. They have proposed that undernutrition at critical points of early fetal development leads to permanent structural and functional changes at later developmental stages and have adverse health outcomes in adulthood.

Neel et al. (1961) proposed the 'thrifty-genotype' hypothesis, which states that an individual's adaptation is due to genes selected over a long period of time.[3] This theory supports the concept of evolutionary enrichment of thrifty genes, i.e., genes that once favored survival during adverse conditions like famine, become detrimental in the later periods of life when food is surplus, thus, increasing disease vulnerability. The behavior of thrifty gene appears to be influenced by the environment to which an individual is exposed.

The 'thrifty phenotype' hypothesis proposed by Hales and Barker (2001) is an alternative to the 'thrifty genotype' and lays emphasis on 'unfavorable intrauterine environment' as an important determinant of adult disease.[4] This was based on an inverse relationship observed between birth weight and risk of type 2 diabetes and metabolic consequences in adulthood.[5]

The two theories that are mentioned above are not mutually exclusive; however, they complement each other. The consequences of both theories are similar, i.e., the adults are well adapted to an environment that is nutritionally limited, but are more likely to become unhealthy in a nutritionally rich environment. It is also clear from the above that certain environmental factors (cues) can induce changes leading to long-term consequences, which manifest as adult diseases.

FETAL PROGRAMMING AND MATERNAL CONSTRAINTS

The consequences of alterations in the developmental environment will depend on how the fetus perceives the environment and responds to it. At certain point of embryonic development, termed as 'critical period', the fetus is capable of adapting to the environmental stress (nutritional and non-nutritional) so as to ensure efficient survival. These adaptive changes termed as 'fetal programming' occur at cellular as well as molecular level. Epigenetic changes, such as DNA methylation, are shown to occur in such stressed fetus resulting in sustained changes in the gene expression.[6] The resultant phenotype is not only expressed in the same individual but is also carried to subsequent generations. The capability of programming extends to a variable period after birth, in infancy, and early childhood. While this adaptation is necessary for the *in utero* survival of the fetus, its continued expression into the postnatal period may actually be disadvantageous. Table 15-1 lists the various prenatal events that can program the developing fetus.

TABLE 15-1

Prenatal Events Leading to Fetal Programming	
• Maternal protein energy malnutrition	• Hypoxia
• Micronutrient deficiencies	• Maternal psychological stress
• Maternal overnutrition and obesity	• Glucocorticoid exposure
• Gestational diabetes mellitus	• Toxins and chemicals
• Infections	

UNDERLYING CAUSAL MECHANISMS

Various causal pathways underlying the associations of birth weight and adult disease have been hypothesized. The proposed theories centrally focus on one of the following:[7-10]

- Fetal undernutrition
- Increased cortisol exposure
- Genetic susceptibility
- Accelerated postnatal growth.

Fetal Undernutrition

Barker's hypothesis provided the first evidence that suboptimal fetal nutrition at critical time period of intrauterine development leads to altered programming.[7,11] Undernutrition of the fetus *in utero* leads to developmental adaptations that permanently alter the fetal structure, function, and metabolism. This results in low birth weight and long-term adverse health outcomes in adulthood. This 'developmental plasticity',—the ability by which an organism adapts itself in response to different environmental cues, may alter programmed growth. This alteration may either favor subsequent growth or may prove detrimental.[12] The growing fetus, which is programmed to suboptimal nutrition from an undernourished mother, exhibits a survival advantage during periods of malnourishment in postnatal life. However, if the same individual is exposed to surplus nutrition in later life, the phenotype changes to a diseased state. Follow-up studies in subjects who have been exposed prenatally to famine during World War II were shown to be associated with coronary heart disease and impaired glucose tolerance in adult life.[13,14] Low birth weight individuals who were reared in affluent countries in later life were shown to develop type 2 diabetes, coronary artery disease, and hypertension.

Most studies that have attempted to explore this hypothesis have relied on birth weight as an important proxy measure for suboptimal growth and development. However, this may not be the causal factor *per se* and other factors that play pivotal role in determining fetal environment and fetal nutrition, such as maternal anthropometrics, maternal diet, and placental function may be strong risk factors for adult disease.

Epidemiological evidence on maternal diet and development of risk factors for cardiovascular disease and type 2 diabetes in adulthood are robust.[13-15] Maternal macro- and micronutrients have shown to be strong determinants of fetal size and health outcomes.[16,17] Results from the Pune Maternal Nutrition study have provided substantial evidence connecting poor nutrition and offspring size in an Indian setting.[18] Rural Indian mothers had a small body frame; consumed low energy and protein, but a higher carbohydrate; and gave birth to babies with relatively lower birth weight compared to mothers in the UK.[19] Analysis of macronutrient intake showed a positive correlation between maternal fat intake at 18 weeks of gestation and fetal size.[20]

Maternal phenotype (prepregnancy body size and metabolic milieu) also appears to be an important determinant for this association. Complications of pregnancy such as preterm delivery, fetal growth restriction due to disorders that cause utero-placental insufficiency, and preeclampsia have been shown to be associated with an increased risk for adult ischemic heart disease, cerebrovascular accidents, and insulin resistance (IR) in later life.[21,22] Maternal and paternal habitus predict offspring's fatness during childhood and altered metabolic sequelae in later life.[23] In all these cases, it is likely that a combination of genetic and environmental factors, operating both pre- and postnatally are important risk determinants.

Steroid Exposure and the Hypothalamic-pituitary-adrenal Axis

Placental glucocorticoid barrier dysfunction leading to increased cortisol exposure is associated with low birth weight and disease in later life.[24] Edwards et al. proposed that absolute or relative impaired activity of placental 11β-hydroxysteroid dehydrogenase (11β-HSD2) associated with an increased maternal cortisol exposes the fetus to excessive cortisol eventually leading to fetal growth retardation, mental retardation, and developmental adaptations that eventually predispose to adult disease.[8] Studies have shown that placental 11β-HSD2 gene expression is impaired in preeclampsia and in low birth weight babies born to maternal pregnancies complicated by eclampsia are born with low birth weight.[25]

An increased cortisol may also be due to developmental changes as a result of various genetic or environmental influences. Lower pituitary-adrenal response to corticotropin-releasing hormone (CRH) stimulation or dexamethasone suppression test [measure of hypothalamic-pituitary-adrenal (HPA) axis] was seen in low birth weight individuals, and provides evidence of dysregulated HPA axis in these individuals.[26] It is however, unclear if increased cortisol exposure is a result of developmental changes in early life or an intermediate in the causal pathway.

The Role of Genes and Environment

The fetal insulin hypothesis by Hattersley and Tooke propose that genetic polymorphisms associated with IR may lead to impaired insulin-mediated growth *in utero* leading to low birth weight and adverse metabolic outcomes in adulthood.[9] Fetal insulin secretion is one of the key determinants of fetal growth, especially in the third trimester. Genetic variants that regulate insulin-mediated fetal growth would also regulate fetal insulin secretion or sensitivity of the fetal tissues to the effects of insulin. This hypothesis provides biological evidence that genetic determinants of birth weight may in addition influence the glucose-insulin homeostasis.

The fetal insulin hypothesis was primarily based on initial studies that demonstrated rare monogenic mutations in the glucokinase gene to be associated with very low birth weight and impaired insulin secretion or insulin sensitivity.[27] Studies on more common genetic variants related to insulin metabolism/impaired glucose tolerance like the insulin gene variable number of tandem repeats (INS VNTR), insulin-like growth factor-1 (IGF-1), and the peroxisome proliferator-activated receptor gamma 2 (PPAR γ2) have demonstrated significant association with low birth weight.[28-30] Recent genome-wide association scans showed strong signals in the adenylate cyclase type 5 (ADCY5) and cyclin L1 (CCNL1) locus to be associated with low birth weight.[31] A longitudinal study from India failed to replicate this finding, but was able to demonstrate genetic variation in the ADCY5 locus to be associated with altered glucose homeostasis, strengthening the link between low birth weight and adult glucose intolerance.[32] It is also important to note that in addition to fetal genetics, maternal and paternal genes may also play an integrated role on the birth weight and adult disease.

Other molecular mechanisms relating to DoHAD include epigenetic currently under investigation include epigenetic modifications leading to permanent inheritable changes in gene expression and mitochondrial dysfunction leading to oxidative damage.[33] The relative contribution of these mechanisms still remains to be established, and extensive studies in the field of epigenetics and fetal origins are believed to provide newer insights into understanding of newer pathways that link birth size and adult disease. Studies in rat models have shown that maternal exposure to low protein diet in pregnancy and lactation results in reduced transcription of hepatocyte nuclear factor-4-α (HNF-4-α) gene in the pancreatic islet cells of the offspring. HNF-4-α is a key transcription factor required for β-cell differentiation and glucose homeostasis. The affected offspring developed diabetes at the age of 17 months substantiating continued expression of the genetic alteration.[34]

While genetic effects on birth weight and adult disease appear to be important, twin studies highlight the importance of environmental influence on genetic variants in disease causation.[35] Reports on monozygotic twins who evolve on a common genetic

TABLE 15-2

Mechanisms of Fetal Programming
• Alterations in cell morphology—pancreatic β-cells, renal nephrons, skeletal myocytes, adipocytes
• Alterations in cellular and hormonal functions—cortisol, insulin, leptin
• Epigenetic changes—methylation, demethylation, and post-translational modification of histone proteins
• Regulation of cell cycle—decreased telomerase activity and accelerated cellular apoptosis during oxidative stress, mitochondrial dysfunction

background, displayed differential weights at birth and developed disease in later life. This clearly strengthens the role of environmental insults over genetic mechanisms.[36-38] Although a similar phenomenon was observed even in discordant twins, conflicting results weakens the hypothesis.

Accelerated Postnatal Growth

Rapid accelerated postnatal growth has been shown to be associated with adult disease.[10] The rapid growth is a common phenomenon observed in many ethnic groups, especially Asians, due to over feeding in the postnatal periods to compensate for the low birth weight. This has been shown to be associated with increased blood pressure, dyslipidemia, obesity, and IR in adulthood. Prospective studies have also shown that weight gain in the first 2 years of life is associated with the development of childhood obesity, independent of birth weight. High body mass index (BMI) in the early childhood in children born with low birth weight leads to impaired IR in adult life.[39,40] Although these evidences favor accelerated growth hypothesis, the association between early weight gain and adult disease may have strong genetic and environmental influences.

Table 15-2 summarizes the cellular alterations during fetal programming.[33]

IMPLICATIONS OF FETAL ORIGINS AND ADULT DISEASE

Numerous diseases associated with low birth weight are listed in table 15-3. The risk for developing disease in adulthood depends on adaptation to transient environmental/nutritional cues exposed during pre- and postnatal life. In the current section, we would briefly discuss evidences favoring the fetal origin of 3 common endocrine disorders, namely type 2 diabetes, obesity, and osteoporosis. The schematic representation of fetal onset of adult diseases has been summarized in figure 15-1.

TABLE 15-3

Adult Diseases Resulting from Fetal Programming	
• Coronary heart disease	• Osteoporosis
• Hypertension	• Psychiatric disorders—depression, anxiety, BPD, schizophrenia
• Hypercholesterolemia	• Alzheimer's disease
• Insulin resistance	• Stroke
• Type 2 diabetes mellitus	• Cancer
• Obesity	• Obstructive lung disease
• Metabolic syndrome	

BPD, borderline personality disorder.

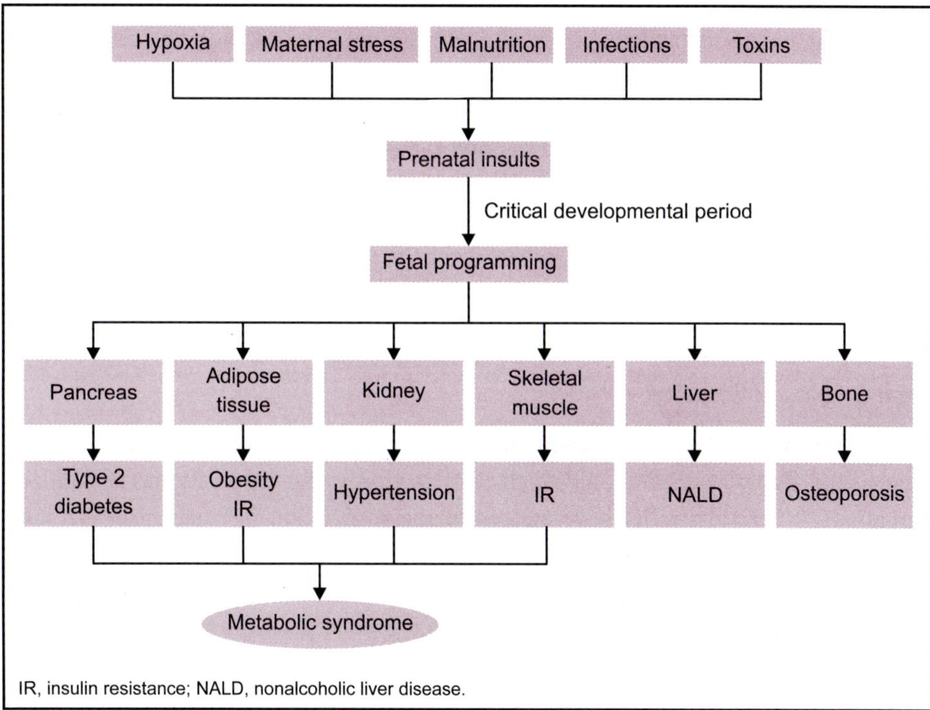

Figure 15-1 A Schematic representation of fetal onset of adult diseases.

Fetal Origins of Type 2 Diabetes

The evidence for association between low birth weight and adult onset hypertension and impaired glucose tolerance is the strongest. Reports on longitudinal follow-up of UK born individuals from 1911–1930 by Hales et al. provided the earliest evidence for the link between lower birth weight and higher rates of type 2 diabetes.[2] This was subsequently confirmed in other large epidemiological cohorts, including the Nurses Health Study. Thinner born babies with low birth size adapt to *in utero* malnutrition through endocrine and metabolic changes leading to IR in childhood and subsequent type 2 diabetes in adulthood.[41,42] Studies from the birth cohort in Mysore, India showed that individuals born with low birth weight were insulin resistant in later life.[43] Yajnik et al. demonstrated a strong relationship between growth velocity in childhood (4–8 years) and adult IR in Indians.[44] Thomas N et al. using hyperinsulinemic-euglycaemic clamp studies, dual energy X-ray absorptiometry, indirect calorimetry, and nuclear magnetic resonance (NMR) spectroscopy, have shown that low weight at birth was associated with changes in diastolic blood pressure and lean body mass. They also showed that in the absence of weight gain, there was minimal impact on glycemic indices by the age of 20 years among rural South Indians.[45] It is important to remember that fetal malnutrition and low birth weight are common among Indians due to chronic undernutrition and high prevalence of anemia in mothers, and this may explain the relatively lower size of Indian babies compared to the West.

While low birth weight is related to adult type 2 diabetes, it is also known that big babies born to women with gestational diabetes are at an additional risk for type 2 diabetes in adulthood. Studies that have explored these 2 aspects have come to the final conclusion that the relationship between birth weight and adult type 2 diabetes is U-shaped.[46,47] The risk of type 2 diabetes in big babies occurs only when the mothers have diabetes during pregnancy.

Fetal Origins of Obesity

The association between birth weight and obesity comes from studies that investigated weight at birth and later BMI, although BMI as a proxy for adiposity has recognized limitations.[48] Several studies have addressed the association of small birth size and subsequent obesity and its metabolic consequences. However, the exact mechanisms of these associations remain elusive. Genetic differences affecting insulin regulation may play a central role as a 'thrifty genotype'.[3,49] This genetic predisposition to nutritional thrift may provide survival advantage for individuals born with lower birth weight. However, as discussed previously, in an environment of excess nutrition, these individuals develop an obese phenotype.

Recently, several possible intrauterine mechanisms that program the infant to central obesity and metabolic syndrome in later life were proposed. Dietary factor appears to be one of the major determinants of fetal programming. Inadequate maternal nutrition and low protein (source of amino acids which are important for the growth and development of pancreatic islets) has been shown to cause permanent changes in the pancreatic vascularity, structure, and functions.[50] Animal models of low protein intake during gestation display long-term changes in pancreatic β-cells and insulin secretion and offspring obesity.[51] Other possible mechanisms, including long-term changes in the activation of the HPA axis, growth hormone, insulin-like growth factors, or sympathetic nervous system have shown to mediate associations between birth weight and later, body proportions.[52,53]

The relationship between birth weight and increased adiposity in later life is also observed among babies born with a higher weight. Results from a large cohort of over 14,000 adolescents in USA have shown that a 1 kg increment in birth weight was associated with an approximately, 50% increase in the risk of overweight at ages 9–14 years, and 30%, when adjusted for maternal BMI.[54] Several factors, such as maternal smoking and socioeconomic status confounds this association. It is unclear if this phenomenon of excess adiposity is consistent across all ethnic groups, since results from some Indian birth cohorts have shown that a low birth weight Indian baby is relatively thin and is more adipose at every ponderal index, and the risk continues throughout life.[55] Therefore, both 'low' and 'high' birth weight Indian babies are at an increased risk for adiposity in adulthood.

Fetal Origins of Osteoporosis

Influence of birth weight on adult bone health is being increasingly appreciated, suggesting a role for fetal programming. Both genetic and epigenetic mechanisms have been shown to be involved in the pathogenesis of osteoporosis resulting from intrauterine programming. Studies have shown that fetus with low birth weight in the presence of polymorphic vitamin D allele develop less adult bone mass.[45,56,58] Furthermore, epigenetic changes have been linked with placental transfer of calcium and vitamin D affecting the fetal bone development and, later, predisposition for adult osteoporosis and osteoarthritis.[57,58]

CONCLUSION

There is now a substantial evidence that favors the relationship between fetal origins and adult diseases. Revolution in the field of genetics and epigenetics may provide more clarity to some of the mechanisms underlying the possible link. This will provide new avenues for early prevention and intervention in reducing the epidemic of noncommunicable diseases.

REFERENCES

1. Barker DJ, Osmond C. Infant mortality, childhood nutrition, and ischaemic heart disease in England and Wales. *Lancet.* 1986;1:1077-81.
2. Hales CN, Barker DJ, Clark PM, Cox LJ, Fall C, Osmond C, et al. Fetal and infant growth and impaired glucose tolerance at age 64. *BMJ.* 1991;303:1019-22.
3. Neel JV. Diabetes mellitus: a "thrifty" genotype rendered detrimental by "progress"? *Am J Hum Genet.* 1962;14:353-62.

4. Hales CN, Barker DJ. The thrifty phenotype hypothesis. *Br Med Bull.* 2001;60:5-20.
5. Gluckman PD, Hanson MA, Beedle AS. Early life events and their consequences for later disease: a life history and evolutionary perspective. *Am J Hum Biol.* 2007;19:1-19.
6. Waterland RA, Michels KB. Epigenetic epidemiology of the developmental origins hypothesis. *Annu Rev Nutr.* 2007;27:363-88.
7. Barker DJ, Gluckman PD, Godfrey KM, Harding JE, Owens JA, Robinson JS. Fetal nutrition and cardiovascular disease in adult life. *Lancet.* 1993;341:938-41.
8. Edwards CR, Benediktsson R, Lindsay RS, Seckl JR. Dysfunction of placental glucocorticoid barrier: link between fetal environment and adult hypertension? *Lancet.* 1993;341:355-7.
9. Hattersley AT, Tooke JE. The fetal insulin hypothesis: an alternative explanation of the association of low birthweight with diabetes and vascular disease. *Lancet.* 1999;353:1789-92.
10. Singhal A, Lucas A. Early origins of cardiovascular disease: is there a unifying hypothesis? *Lancet.* 2004;363:1642-5.
11. Barker DJ. Fetal origins of coronary heart disease. *BMJ.* 1995;311:171-4.
12. Bateson, P, Barker D, Clutton-Brock T, Deb D, D'Udine B, Foley RA, et al. Developmental plasticity and human health. *Nature.* 2004;430:419-21.
13. Ravelli AC, van der Menlen JH, Michels RP, Osmond C, Barker DJ, Hales CN, et al. Glucose tolerance in adults after prenatal exposure to famine. *Lancet.* 1998;351:173-7.
14. Roseboom TJ, van der Menlen JH, Osmond C, Barker DJ, Ravelli AC, Schroeder-Tanka JM, et al. Coronary heart disease after prenatal exposure to the Dutch famine. 1944–45. *Heart.* 2000;84:595-8.
15. Stanner SA, Bulmer K, Andres C, Lantseva OE, Borodina V, Poteen W. Does malnutrition in utero determine diabetes and coronary heart disease in adulthood? Results from the Leningrad siege study, a cross sectional study. *BMJ.* 1997;315:1342-8.
16. Campbell DM, Hall MH, Barker DJ, Cross J, Shiell AW, Godfrey KM. Diet in pregnancy and the offspring's blood pressure 40 years later. *Br J Obstet Gynaecol.*1996;103:273-80.
17. Shiell AW, Campbell-Brown M, Haselden S, Robinson S, Godfrey KM, Barker DJ. High-meat, low-carbohydrate diet in pregnancy: relation to adult blood pressure in the offspring. *Hypertension.* 2001;38:1282-8.
18. Yajnik CS, Fall CH, Coyaja KJ, Hirve SS, Rao S, Barker DJ, et al. Neonatal anthropometry: the thin-fat Indian baby. The Pune Maternal Nutrition Study. *Int J Obes Relat Metab Disord.* 2003;27:173-80.
19. Rao S, Yajnik CS, Kanada A, Fall CH, Margetts BM, Jackson AA, et al. Intake of micronutrient-rich foods in rural Indian mothers is associated with the size of their babies at birth: Pune Maternal Nutrition Study. *J Nutr.* 2001;131:1217-24.
20. Shiell AW, Campbell Dm, Hall MH, Barker DJ. Diet in late pregnancy and glucose-insulin metabolism of the offspring 40 years later. *BJOG.* 2000;107:890-5.
21. Pell JP, Smith GC, Walsh D. Pregnancy complications and subsequent maternal cerebrovascular events: a retrospective cohort study of 119,668 births. *Am J Epidemiol.* 2004;159: 336-42.
22. Smith GC, Pell JP, Walsh D. Pregnancy complications and maternal risk of ischaemic heart disease: a retrospective cohort study of 129,290 births. *Lancet.* 2001;357:2002-6.
23. Lindsay RS, Dabelea D, Roumain J, Hanson RL, Benett PH, Knowler WC. Type 2 diabetes and low birth weight: the role of paternal inheritance in the association of low birth weight and diabetes. *Diabetes.* 2000;49:445-9.

24. Seckl JR. Prenatal glucocorticoids and long-term programming. *Eur J Endocrinol.* 2004;151: U49-62.
25. Schoof E, Girstl M, Frobenins W, Kirschbaum M, Dorr HG, Rascher W, et al. Decreased gene expression of 11beta-hydroxysteroid dehydrogenase type 2 and 15-hydroxyprostaglandin dehydrogenase in human placenta of patients with preeclampsia. *J Clin Endocrinol Metab.* 2001;86:1313-7.
26. Ward AM, Syddall HE, Wood PJ, Chrousos GP, Phillips DI. Fetal programming of the hypothalamic-pituitary-adrenal (HPA) axis: low birth weight and central HPA regulation. *J Clin Endocrinol Metab.* 2004;89:1227-33.
27. Weedon MN, Frayling TM, Shields B, Knight B, Turner T, Metcalf BS, et al. Genetic regulation of birth weight and fasting glucose by a common polymorphism in the islet cell promoter of the glucokinase gene. *Diabetes.* 2005;54:576-81.
28. Andersson EA, Pilqaard K, Pisinger C, Harder MN, Grarup N, Faerch K, et al. Type 2 diabetes risk alleles near ADCY5, CDKAL1 and HHEX-IDE are associated with reduced birthweight. *Diabetologia.* 2010;53:1908-16.
29. Lindsay RS, Hanson RL, Wiedrich C, Knowler WC, Bennett PH, Baier LJ. The insulin gene variable number tandem repeat class I/III polymorphism is in linkage disequilibrium with birth weight but not Type 2 diabetes in the Pima population. *Diabetes.* 2003;52:187-93.
30. Vaessen N, Janssen JA, Hentink P, Hofman A, Lamberts SW, Oostra BA, et al. Association between genetic variation in the gene for insulin-like growth factor-I and low birthweight. *Lancet.* 2002;359:1036-7.
31. Freathy RM, Mook-Kanamori DO, Sovio U, Prokopenko I, Timpson NJ, Berry DJ, et al. Variants in ADCY5 and near CCNL1 are associated with fetal growth and birth weight. *Nat Genet.* 2010;42:430-5.
32. Vasan SK, Neville MJ, Antonisawy B, Samuel P, Fall CH, Geethanjali FS, et al. Absence of birth-weight lowering effect of ADCY5 and near CCNL, but association of impaired glucose-insulin homeostasis with ADCY5 in Asian Indians. *PLoS One.* 2011;6:e21331.
33. Warner MJ, Ozanne SE. Mechanisms involved in the developmental programming of adulthood disease. *Biochem J.* 2010;427:333-47.
34. Sandovici I, Smith NH, Nitert MD, Ackers-Johnson M, Uribe-Lewis S, Ito Y, et al. Maternal diet and aging alter the epigenetic control of a promoter–enhancer interaction at the Hnf4a gene in rat pancreatic islets. *Proc Natl Acad Sci USA.* 2011;108:5449-54.
35. Hubinette A, Cnattingius S, Ekbam A, de Faire U, Kramer M, Lichtenstein P. Birthweight, early environment, and genetics: a study of twins discordant for acute myocardial infarction. *Lancet.* 2001;357:1997-2001.
36. Baird J, Osmond C, MacGregor A, Snieder H, Hales CN, Philips DI. Testing the fetal origins hypothesis in twins: the Birmingham twin study. *Diabetologia.* 2001;44:33-9.
37. Iliadou A, Cnattingius S, Lichtenstein P. Low birthweight and Type 2 diabetes: a study on 11 162 Swedish twins. *Int J Epidemiol.* 2004;33:948-53.
38. Poulsen P, Vaag AA, Kwik KO, Moller Jensen D, Beck-Nielsen H. Low birth weight is associated with NIDDM in discordant monozygotic and dizygotic twin pairs. *Diabetologia.* 1997;40:439-46.
39. Ong KK, Ahmed ML, Emmett PM, Preece MA, Dunger DB. Association between postnatal catch-up growth and obesity in childhood: prospective cohort study. *BMJ.* 2000;320:967-71.

40. Stettler N, Zemel BS, Kumanyika S, Stallings VA. Infant weight gain and childhood overweight status in a multicenter, cohort study. *Pediatrics*. 2002;109:194-9.
41. Lithell HO, McKeique PM, Berghend L, Mohsen R, Lithel UB, Lem DA. Relation of size at birth to non-insulin dependent diabetes and insulin concentrations in men aged 50-60 years. *BMJ*. 1996;312:406-10.
42. Phillips DI. Insulin resistance as a programmed response to fetal undernutrition. *Diabetologia*. 1996;39:1119-22.
43. Fall CH, Stein CE, Kumaran K, Cox V, Osmond C, Baker DJ, et al. Size at birth, maternal weight, and type 2 diabetes in South India. *Diabet Med*. 1998;15:220-7.
44. Yajnik CS. Nutrition, growth, and body size in relation to insulin resistance and type 2 diabetes. *Curr Diab Rep*. 2003;3:108-14.
45. Thomas N, Grunnet G, Pouben P, Christopher S, Spongem R, Irbakumari M, et al. Born With Low Birth Weight in Rural Southern India - What Are the Metabolic Consequences 20 Years Later? *Eur J Endocrinol*. 2012;166:647-55.
46. Rich-Edwards JW, Colditz GA, Stampfer MJ, Willet WC, Gillman MW, Hennekens CH, et al. Birthweight and the risk for type 2 diabetes mellitus in adult women. *Ann Intern Med*. 1999;130:278-84.
47. Yajnik CS. The insulin resistance epidemic in India: fetal origins, later lifestyle, or both? *Nutr Rev*. 2001;59:1-9.
48. Oken E, Gillman MW. Fetal origins of obesity. *Obes Res*. 2003;11:496-506.
49. Bhargava SK, Sachdev HS, Fall CH, Osmond C, Lakshay R, Barker DJ, et al. Relation of serial changes in childhood body-mass index to impaired glucose tolerance in young adulthood. *N Engl J Med*. 2004;350:865-75.
50. Hales CN, Barker DJ. Type 2 (non-insulin-dependent) diabetes mellitus: the thrifty phenotype hypothesis. *Diabetologia*. 1992;35:595-601.
51. Petry CJ, Ozanne SE, Hales CN. Programming of intermediary metabolism. *Mol Cell Endocrinol*. 2001;185:81-91.
52. Flanagan DE, Moore VM, Godsland IF, Cockington RA, Robinson JS, Phillips DI. Reduced foetal growth and growth hormone secretion in adult life. *Clin Endocrinol (Oxf)*. 1999;50: 735-40.
53. Phillips DI, Barker DJ. Association between low birthweight and high resting pulse in adult life: is the sympathetic nervous system involved in programming the insulin resistance syndrome? *Diabet Med*. 1997;14:673-7.
54. Gillman MW, Rifas-Shiman S, Berkey CS, Field AE, Colditz GA. Maternal gestational diabetes, birth weight, and adolescent obesity. *Pediatrics*. 2003;111:e221-6.
55. Joglekar CV, Fall CH, Deshpande VIJ, Joshi N, Balerao A, Solat V, et al. Newborn size, infant and childhood growth, and body composition and cardiovascular disease risk factors at the age of 6 years: the Pune Maternal Nutrition Study. *Int J Obes (Lond)*. 2007;31:1534-44.
56. Keen RW, Egger P, Fall C, Major PJ, Lanchbury JS, Spector TD, et al. Polymorphisms of the vitamin D receptor, infant growth, and adult bone mass. *Calcif Tissue Int*. 1997;60:233-5.
57. Bocheva G, Boyadjieva N. Epigenetic regulation of fetal bone development and placental transfer of nutrients: progress for osteoporosis. *Interdiscip Toxicol*. 2011;4:167-72.
58. Antoniades L, MacGregor AJ, Andrew T, Spector TD. Association of Osteoporosis and Osteoarthritis in adult twins. *Rheumatology*. 2003;42:791-6.

Index

Page numbers followed by *f* refer to figure and *t* refer to table.

A

Abdominal pain 126
Abnormal glucose tolerance 13
Abruptio placenta 85
Accelerated postnatal growth 153, 156
Acromegaly 108
Activated partial thromboplastin time 82
Acute pulmonary edema 85
Adrenal
  cortex 71
  disorders in pregnancy 118
  functions during pregnancy 118
  glands 7
  insufficiency 120
Adrenocorticotropic hormone 2, 71, 106
Alanine transaminase 80
Aldosterone 2
Alzheimer's disease 157
American
  Academy of Pediatrics 20
  Association of Clinical Endocrinologists 41
  Congress of Obstetricians and Gynecologist 18, 41, 147
  Diabetes Association 14, 16
  Heart Association 140
  Society for Reproductive Medicine 131
  Thyroid Association 40
Anencephaly 12
Angiotensin converting enzyme inhibitors 20, 83
Anterior pituitary disorders 108
Antidiuretic hormone 6
Antithyroid drugs 47
Arginine vasopressin 6
Aspartate transaminase 80
Assessment of iodine status during pregnancy 30
Asthma 89
Atlantic Diabetes in Pregnancy 141
Atrial septal defect 12
Autism 89
Autoimmune thyroid disorders and pregnancy 38

B

Bacterial vaginosis 89
Biochemical signs of hyperandrogenism 131
Bipedal edema 126
Blood glucose 126
Body mass index 82, 139, 156
Bone disorders and pregnancy 96
Borderline personality disorder 157

C

Calcitonin 98, 99
Calcium 96, 98
  ions 59
  metabolism during
    lactation 98
    pregnancy 58, 59*f*, 96
  sarcoplasmic reticulum 59
Cancer 157

Cardiac anomalies 12
Caudal regression 12
Central nervous system 145
Cesarean section 142
Chronic hypertension 79, 82
Chvostek's sign 63
Classification of hypertensive disorders during pregnancy 80*t*
Clomiphene citrate 109, 134
Clonidine 84
Congenital adrenal hyperplasia 122, 123, 131
Contraception 146
Coronary heart disease 157
Corticotropin releasing hormone 2, 105, 154
Cushing's
  disease 110, 111
  syndrome 110, 111, 119
Cystic kidney 12

D

Definition of preeclampsia 80
Deoxycorticosterone 2
Development of eclampsia 85*t*
Developmental origins of health and disease 151
Dexamethasone suppression test 154
Diabetes
  insipidus 115
  mellitus 157
Diastolic blood pressure 80
Disorders of bone metabolism 100
Dual-energy x-ray absorptiometry 99

E

Endocrinology of hyperemesis gravidarum 66
Estriol 2
Estrogen 3, 37, 69
European Society of Human Reproduction and Embryology 131

F

Familial hypocalciuric hypercalcemia 61
Fasting glucose concentration 15
Fetal
  and neonatal consequences of maternal hypothyroidism 37
  heart rate 54
  intrauterine growth retardation 14
  neonatal consequences of maternal iodine deficiency 28
  origins of
    endocrine disease 151
    obesity 158
    osteoporosis 159
    type 2 diabetes 157
  skeletal disorders 89
  thyroid physiology 46
  undernutrition 153
Follicle stimulating hormone 5, 107
Free thyroxine 37
Function of corpus luteum 3

G

Gastrointestinal dysfunction 71
Gestational
  diabetes mellitus 13-16, 89, 136, 139, 142, 144, 153
    diagnostic criteria 15, 16*t*
  hypertension 79, 80*t*
  thyrotoxicosis 50
  trophoblastic disease 82
  weight gain recommendations 140*t*
Glomerular filtration rate 26, 36, 98
Glucocorticoid exposure 153
Gonadotropin
  axis 107
  releasing hormone 2, 134
Graves' disease 48, 49, 52, 53, 55, 56, 70
Growth hormone 2, 4, 106, 145
  releasing hormone 2

H

Headache 126
Helicobacter pylori infection 69
HELLP syndrome 115

Hepatic dysfunction 71
Human
  chorionic gonadotropin 2, 3, 37, 47, 50, 67, 68, 106
  immunodeficiency virus 89
  placental lactogen 2, 3, 14, 88, 136
Hydatidiform mole 49
Hydralazine 84
Hydrocortisone 114
Hydrops fetalis 82
Hyperacuity of olfactory system 72
Hypercalcemia during pregnancy 61
Hypercholesterolemia 157
Hyperemesis gravidarum 49, 73
Hypertension 79, 85, 126, 157
Hypertensive disorders of pregnancy 142
Hyperthyroidism 54
Hypothyroidism 36
Hypoparathyroidism 63, 101
Hypophysitis 111, 112*f*
Hypopituitarism 112
Hypothalamic pituitary-adrenal axis 106, 118, 154
Hypoxia 153

I

Implications of
  fetal origins and adult disease 156
  vitamin D deficiency in female reproduction 90
In vitro fertilization 89, 124, 135
Indian Thyroid Society 33, 40, 43, 53, 54
Indications of delivery in women with preeclampsia and gestational hypertension 85*t*
Inferior petrosal venous sinus sampling 111
Infertility 90, 133
Insulin 18
  like growth factor-1 5, 108
    binding protein type-1 134
  pump 19
  resistance 8, 14, 92, 157
  sensitivity 14
Intrauterine growth retardation 61, 79, 85, 120
Iodine 37
  induced hyperthyroidism 49
  metabolism in pregnancy 24, 25
  physiology 25
  supplementation 30
    during pregnancy 29

K

Ketamine 85
Ketoconazole 111

L

Labetalol 84
Lactate dehydrogenase 80
Lactotroph hypertrophy 105
Laparoscopic ovarian drilling 135
Leptin 70
Levothyroxine 40, 43
Liver transaminases 126
Low density lipoprotein 2, 132
Lower
  bone mineral density 96
  esophageal sphincter pressure 68
Luteinizing hormone 3, 107, 134
Lymphocyte infiltration 112*f*

M

Magnetic resonance imaging 4, 102
Management of
  infertility in PCOS 133
  postpartum thyroiditis 43*t*
  thyrotoxicosis during pregnancy 54*t*
Maternal
  and placental adrenocorticotropic hormone 118
  fetal HIV transfer 89
  low-density lipoprotein 2
  morbidity 141
  overnutrition and obesity 153
  plasma concentration 3
  protein energy malnutrition 153

psychological stress 153
thyroid physiology in pregnancy 46
Mean plasma glucose 17
Measuring blood pressure during pregnancy 81*t*
Mechanisms of fetal programming 156*t*
Medical nutrition therapy 17
Metabolic syndrome 157
Methimazole 52
Methyldopa 84
Micronutrient deficiencies 153
Microvascular disease 82
Migraine 82
Mild hypertension 80
Moderate hypertension 80
Multiple
gestations 73, 82
sclerosis 89

N

National
High Blood Pressure Education Program 79
Institute for Health and Clinical Excellence 85, 86
Nausea 66
Neonatal hypocalcemia and seizures 89
Neural tube defects 12
Neutral protamine hagedorn 19
Nifedipine 84
Nonalcoholic
fatty liver disease 145
liver disease 157
Nonfunctioning adenomas 111
Non-reassuring fetal status 85
Nonsteroidal anti-inflammatory drugs 85
Nuclear magnetic resonance 158

O

Obesity 82, 146, 157
and pregnancy 139
Obstructive lung disease 157
Oral glucose tolerance test 16, 109
Orthostatic hypotension 126
Osteoporosis 157
in pregnancy 102

P

Pancreas 8
Parathyroid
disorders during pregnancy 58
glands 7
hormone 59, 96, 98, 99
plasma concentrations 7
related peptide 98, 99
related protein 2
Pathogenesis of hyperemesis gravidarum 68*f*
Pathophysiology of hyperemesis gravidarum 67
Perinatal
morbidity 142
mortality 137
Persistent epigastric pain 85
Pheochromocytoma 125, 126*t*
Phosphate ions 59
Pituitary
adenoma 108*f*
disorders in pregnancy 105
gland 4, 105, 105*f*
gonadotropins 107
growth hormone 106
Placental
corticotropin releasing hormone 118
transport of thyroid hormones 47*f*
Plasma
inorganic iodide 25, 28
renin activity 118
Polycystic ovarian syndrome 89, 91, 131
Posterior pituitary 108
disorders 114
Postpartum
depression 42
hypercalcemia 61
thyroiditis 42, 42*t*, 49
Prazosin 84
Prednisolone 114

Preeclampsia 89, 126*t*
Pre-existing hypertension 80
Pregestational diabetes 12
Pregnancy
  and diabetes mellitus 12
  induced hypertension 137
  related hypertension 137
Premature rupture of membranes 18
Primary hyperparathyroidism 59, 60, 100
Progesterone 2, 68
Prolactin 4, 5*f*, 68, 105
  axis 106
Prolactinomas 109
Propylthiouracil 54
Pseudohypoparathyroidism 101

R

Rectal atresia 12
Red blood cells 82
Renal
  anomalies 12
  disease 82
Renin angiotensin-aldosterone system 108
Role of
  glucose monitoring 19
  iodine nutrition in pregnancy 27

S

Salt fortification with iodine 29
Schizophrenia 89
Serum prolactin 105
Severe fetal IUGR 85
Sex hormone-binding globulin 8, 134
Sheehan's syndrome 113
Situs inversus 12
Somatostatin 2
Spina bifida 12
Spontaneous preterm birth 89
Steroid exposure and hypothalamic-pituitary-adrenal axis 154
Stroke 157
Subacute thyroiditis 49
Subclassification of hypertension during pregnancy 80*t*
Systemic lupus erythematosus 82
Systolic blood pressure 80

T

Tamoxifen 135
Thrombocytopenia 126
Thrombophilia 82
Thyroglobulin 28, 32, 37
Thyroid
  autoimmunity in pregnancy 47
  binding globulin 36, 37
  function in iodine deficient states 28*f*
  gland 6
  hormone 67, 70
  peroxidase antibody 37, 40, 42, 43
  related changes in pregnancy 47*t*
  stimulating hormone 26, 32, 38, 40, 54, 67, 106
    receptor antibody 54
  storm 55
  surgery 53
  stimulating hormone 28, 37, 43, 47, 51
    receptor antibody 47, 51
Thyroperoxidase 25
Thyrotoxicosis in pregnancy 46
Thyrotropin releasing hormone 2, 106
Thyroxine 37, 40, 47, 49, 54, 68
  binding globulin 6, 47, 106
Total parathyroid hormone 59
Toxic
  adenoma 49
  multinodular goiter 49
Transposition of great vessel 12
Treatment of
  hypertension in pregnancy 84*t*
  hypopituitarism in pregnancy 113, 114*t*
Triiodothryonine 28, 40, 47, 49, 68
Trophoblastic disease 73
  of pregnancy 49
Trousseau's sign 63
Tyrosine residues of thyroglobulin 25

U

Ureter duplex 12*t*
Urinary iodine concentration 30, 31

V

Vestibular disorders 72
Vitamin D 90, 98, 99
  and fertility 90
  and fetal programming 92
  and hypertensive disorders in pregnancy 91
  and mode of delivery 91
  and other pregnancy-associated disorders 92
  and pregnancy 88
  and spontaneous preterm birth 91
  deficiency on maternal and fetal health 89*t*
  metabolism in pregnancy 88
  supplementation in pregnancy 92
Vomiting 66

W

White classification of diabetes during pregnancy 13*t*
World Health Organization 16